Managing Your Career in Nursing

Managing Your Career in Nursing

Frances C. Henderson, RN, EdD
Professor and Chairperson
Department of Baccalaureate Nursing
Alcorn State University
Natchez, Mississippi

Barbara O. McGettigan, RN, MS
Assistant Director of Educational Services
Children's Hospital
San Francisco, California

ADDISON-WESLEY PUBLISHING COMPANY
Reading, Massachusetts · Menlo Park, California
Don Mills, Ontario · Wokingham, England · Amsterdam
Sydney · Singapore · Tokyo · Madrid · Bogotá
Santiago · San Juan

Sponsoring Editor: Nancy Evans
Production Supervisor: Anne Friedman
Interior Designer: Richard Kharibian
Cover Designer: John Osborne
Copyeditor: Helene Harrington

Library of Congress Cataloging-in-Publication Data

Henderson, Frances C.
  Managing your career in nursing.

  Bibliography: p.
  Includes index.
  1. Nursing—Vocational guidance.   I. McGettigan,
Barbara O.   II. Title.   [DNLM: 1. Career Mobility.
2. Nursing.   WY 16 H496m]
RT82.H46   1986   610.73'023   86-17396
ISBN 0-201-12958-2

  CDEFGHIJ-AL-8987

Addison-Wesley Publishing Company
Health Sciences Division
2725 Sand Hill Road
Menlo Park, California 94025

Contents

Foreword

At last, here is a book to convince us that it is not only possible but essential to *manage* a career in nursing, a concept that has been clear for some time to those in other professions. And, at last, we have a valuable resource to use in counseling those who are groping their way through career dilemmas.

Managing Your Career in Nursing by Henderson and McGettigan will be a welcome addition to every nurse's personal library—a book we will want to be introduced to as students and to keep around for periodic referral during our lifetime. It guides us in thinking about our professional goals and choosing a pathway for ourselves within the larger context of health and social forces.

The authors tantalize us with the prospect of attaining and maintaining career vitality, manifested in enjoying our work, believing our work makes a contribution to society, and seeing a balance between rewards and effort. Then we proceed through a step-by-step process involving assessment of ourselves, professional options, and current trends. The pages thus become a chronicle of personal aspiration, appraisal, and commitment—commitment to creating our own destiny.

Margretta M. Styles
President
American Nurses' Association
Professor
School of Nursing
University of California, San Francisco

Preface

The expansion of nursing options, evidenced by changes in nurses' practice settings and scope of responsibilities, requires that nurses set clear professional goals. Nurses must use effective career management strategies to maximize their personal growth while contributing to the integrity and growth of the profession. Our principal goal is to provide nurses with a practical, self-directed approach for lifelong career management. Using this approach, nurses can increase professional and career autonomy, face personal and professional transitions confidently, and enhance career satisfaction and vitality within the context of nursing, societal, and health care trends.

Range of Uses

This book serves as a mentor-in-print whether you are a beginning student in a nursing education program or one who is about to graduate, a registered nurse enrolled in a baccalaureate or higher degree program, or a nurse in clinical practice considering career ladder opportunities, role expansion, or exploring career issues.

Managing Your Career in Nursing can be used as a textbook for courses in career management and professional nursing roles or as a supplement to courses focusing on nursing trends, staff development, and professional issues. Its use can range from self-directed independent study to large group study with an instructor. Preceptors, staff development specialists, faculty, and nurse advisors may also use it in informal career development seminars. Additionally, this book can be used as a reference by non-nurses who provide career guidance to nurses and aspiring nursing students.

Key Features

The guidebook format is designed to engage you in a personal and professional developmental process that will:
—help you find answers to your career management questions,
—empower you to validate previous decisions, choices, and strategies, and
—help you shape your career future.

This book goes beyond traditional discussions of nursing options and roles. It is based on our career management framework which encompasses the self, nursing options and trends, and key career management strategies. By analyzing various dimensions of practice, you can develop a solid basis for establishing career goals that match personal characteristics, attributes, style, and stage. You can go beyond a single job outlook to a professional career perspective. And by learning methods for examining trends, you can approach career planning from a lifelong perspective.

The focus of this book is the why, what, and how of career management for nurses. The first three chapters give you an overview of rationale, characteristics, and a framework of career management. Chapter 4 provides you with strategies and resources for gathering information. Chapters 5, 6, and 7 guide you in assessing yourself, nursing options, and trends, while Chapter 8 provides guidelines for choosing career goals and making a career plan. Chapter 9 includes four key strategies for effective career management. In this book you will systematically assess and evaluate, make and implement career plans to reach specific career goals. In addition, you will apply problem solving and other strategies to managing your career.

The subjects within each chapter are presented with illustrations, case examples, and comments from the nursing literature. A variety of exercises and activities guides you in applying the career management process. Although we recommend you complete all exercises, they may not all appeal to you; if so, you can choose to complete summary exercises or selected ones that best meet your needs.

Two other features of this book are its versatility and its self-directed approach. You can use it as a reference for selected career concerns or read it from cover to cover. Since career management is lifelong, you can periodically review selected sections, redo exercises, and update your career planning portfolio as indicated by personal and career changes. The self-directed approach of this book is intended to guide *you* in exploring those essential components and strategies necessary for managing *your* career in nursing.

Frances C. Henderson
Barbara O. McGettigan

Acknowledgments

The process of writing this book was the achievement of a mutually held and highly valued goal. In so doing over the past four years we have experienced personal and professional growth. Its publication and our anticipation of its usefulness to you in career management will perpetually inspire our career vitality.

We would like to express our appreciation to a number of special people who helped us to transform our dream into the reality you now hold in your hand.

Cecelia Dwydiak, Marjorie Habeeb, Estrella Manio, and Marilyn Rajokovich shared time and energy in early discussions and planning about the career management resources needed by nurses.

Students, nurses in clinical practice, nursing educators, and others involved with a variety of aspects of nursing shared invaluable insights into the demands and expectations, joys, and terrors of nursing career dilemmas. In so doing they fueled our creative energy.

Nancy Evans, our editor, and the staff at Addison–Wesley were invaluable sources of patience, guidance, support, print media, and other resources.

Judith Spencer used her talents as writer, thinker, referee, and freelance developmental editor to bring us over many hurdles and helped hone our drafts into a presentable manuscript.

Our faithful and patient manuscript typist, Debra Trulin, made our handwritten symbols come alive on typewritten pages. Hers was a difficult task with tight deadlines and large volumes of work. Hedy Arterburn, Peggy Crain, and Ann Zapponi also helped with typing portions of the manuscript.

Three freelance artists helped us with the early phases of developing illustrations. Bob Spencer, Rebecca Varella, and Anne Batmale.

We highly value our reviewers who were as free with their compliments as they were with their critiques:

Nancy Diekelmann, PhD, RN, FAAN, University of Wisconsin, Madison,

WI; Cynthia M. Freund, PhD, RN, University of North Carolina, Chapel Hill, NC; Barbara Huttman, MS, RN, San Francisco Children's Hospital, CA; Phyllis Irvine, PhD, RN, Northeastern Louisiana University, LA; Janice Bell Meisenhelder, DNSc, Northeastern University, MA; Patricia Moccia, PhD, RN, Columbia University, NY; Belinda Puetz, PhD, RN, Continuing Education Unlimited, Indianapolis, IN; Delight M. Tillotson, MSN, RN, University of Texas, San Antonio, TX; Connie Vance, EdD, RN, New York University, NY.

Margretta Styles, whose book *On Nursing: Toward a New Endowment,* provided us with much inspiration, has honored us by writing the foreword.

Our friends who understood the constraints on our time for socializing were most supportive and encouraging.

And to our families. Only a special loving husband like Neal McGettigan could adapt so well for so long. Cynthia, Don, and Steven Henderson, sensitive and supportive, were always encouraging and empathetic. We share with you not only the reward of more of our time but our pride in the finished product.

We acknowledge each other for neither of us could have achieved this goal alone.

F.C.H.
B.O.M.

1 Why Career Management?

FRANCES C. HENDERSON
BARBARA O. McGETTIGAN

Many career dilemmas that relate to both professional and societal changes face nurses today. New expectations for nursing education and practice combine with upheavals in the nature, structure, and management of work and with gender-related issues to evoke nurses' concerns about career and career management. In today's environment nurses often experience career transitions and role stress. Simultaneously, nurses seek career vitality, a sense of fulfillment, in their practice of nursing. Seeking career vitality, coping with role stress, and addressing career concerns all support the critical need for effective career management.

This chapter explores societal and professional changes that will enable you to broaden your perspective when addressing your career and its dilemmas. This chapter also describes common nurses' career syndromes and characteristics of career vitality. You will have an opportunity to assess your current experiences with career stress and level of vitality. We hope you will achieve a sense of support knowing that your career concerns and experiences are phenomena shared by many nurses and members of the workplace. We start by taking a closer look at some of the major professional and societal changes that make career management an essential survival skill for you.

Professional Changes

Educational requirements and definitions of nursing practice are among the signposts of our evolving profession. Although exciting and challenging, these professional developments make career management imperative and cause nurses to raise questions such as the following:

1. If I want to go into nursing administration, should I get a master's degree in nursing, in business, or both?

2. If I choose oncology nursing, will I be able to make a change to another specialty?

3. If I choose to be a nurse practitioner, will I be marketable and in what settings?

4. I would like to run the nursing services of a home health agency. Do I need to work in a hospital first, or is there a ladder in such agencies?

5. I think I'd like to be a clinical nurse specialist but I'm not sure there will be a place for such a role in a prospective payment system (PPS).

6. Can I get academic credit toward my BSN for achieving certification in neurosurgical nursing?

Have you raised these or similar questions? Take a moment now to write your own questions or dilemmas related to professional changes.

_____

_____

_____

Frequently asked questions like these reflect the still evolving nature of the nursing profession. These questions symbolize the growing pains of a profession steeped in tradition, influenced by stereotypes, but reaching toward theory building and responding to consumer health needs and demands. Appreciating this stage of development in both nursing education and practice helps you answer questions, deal with dilemmas, and recognize why career management is imperative.

Nursing Education

At all levels of nursing, educational requirements are changing. In 1985 the House of Delegates of the American Nurses' Association (ANA) voted decisively that the title Registered Nurse (RN) should be reserved for the professional nurse prepared at the baccalaureate level with a major in nursing. They also voted that the title Associate Nurse would refer to a technical nurse educated in associate degree programs in institutions of higher education (AJN, 1985). At advanced levels of practice, such as nursing specialization, the ANA Social Policy Statement (1980) recommends the Master of Science degree (MSN) in nursing. The need for doctoral level preparation in nursing is increasing for nursing research, administration, and education.

Increasing complexities in nursing practice demand lifelong formal and informal education. Expanding roles in clinics, home care, community-based mental health services, adult day care, and geriatric care require education for independent or collaborative practice. Sophisticated technical and psychosocial aspects of acute care necessitate special education, certification, and advanced nursing degrees. For management positions, such as head nurse and supervisor, minimal educational requirements are BSN and in many cases an MSN is preferred. Deciding about educational advancement is a growing concern for many nurses. Making education-related decisions is only a part of the career management process.

Nursing Practice

An environment of competitive and limited health care resources is propelling nurses to clearly define their practice, function, and role in the health care system. The profession's current definition of nursing reflects a shift in emphasis from *care* to *diagnosis,* from *actions* to *treatment,* and from *patient* to *client.* These words convey the development of more independent, accountable, and collaborative practice. Reaching beyond the challenge of defining nursing to marketing and receiving adequate reimbursement for nursing service are major career management concerns.

Nursing roles, such as clinical nurse specialist and nurse practitioner, are expanding beyond mere extensions into medical arenas to more sophisticated and autonomous functions. Expertise in patient care management is no longer enough for head nurses and nursing service directors. Nurse managers develop and monitor budgets, manage people, and participate in strategic planning and new product development. Staff nurses are expanding their functions to include coordinating client care, planning discharges, implementing client teaching, and providing home-liaison services. Opportunities for specialists and nurse practitioners are available in primary care, health promotion, rehabilitation, and geriatrics.

When you assess, plan, and manage your career, you can take better advantage of opportunities presented by these new or changing roles. A well-designed plan and use of career management strategies can help you anticipate and deal with these changes.

Changes in nursing education and nursing practice are greatly influenced by broad societal changes. These societal changes reflect the effects of the past on the present as well as the influence of new technologies, theories, and values. An overview of some societal changes further elaborates the complexity and salience of career concerns and the relevance of effective career management.

Societal Changes

Societal changes related to both work and gender influence nurses' careers, experiences, and strategies. New directions in the nature of work as well as the structure and management of work have a far-reaching effect on careers. Gender-related issues also support the value of career management for nurses.

Since nursing is predominantly a female profession, beliefs about working women and the effects of socialization, stereotypes, and barriers on careers can needlessly hamper nurses' career advancement.

Work-Related Changes

Changes in the level and type of work, the profile of the worker, and the workplace require a new interpretation of career and emphasize the need for clear goals and fine skills in career management. These work-related changes necessitate a shift in perspective from career as a stable, lifelong job in a single organization to career as a pattern of varying types of work within complex and changing organizations. The individual adapts within this dynamic environment of work if anchored by clear career goals, possessed of broad, transferrable skills, cognizant of trends, and directed by a plan.

Nature of Work and the Work Force. The knowledge explosion and high technology have combined with demographics and shifts in life values to create profound upheavals in the nature of work and the work force. Certain jobs have become obsolete, resulting in worker displacement. Job loss causes lowered self-esteem and depression, which can further limit job access. While some jobs have diminished, the need for computer programmers, technicians, telecommunicators, and information managers has escalated. Preparing for these types of jobs can cause personal strain or satisfaction.

The profile of the worker is changing. The general population is older; those who are age 65 have 12 or more years of living ahead of them. A longer life span presents various career options. It may mean longer length of employment, a combination of part-time work for pay and nonpaying work, or it may mean a shift entirely to other life activities. Those seeking promotion in the 35 to 45-year-old group may find fewer openings because of the increased numbers in the 50 to 70-year-old group who are retaining their positions. This may cause frustrations or stimulate exploration of other options such as lateral moves or independent business.

In addition to changes in life span, the population is becoming more knowledgeable, advancing in educational preparation. We see full professors after 6 to 10 years in the academic setting and increasing numbers of persons at the doctorate level in all general job levels. Advances in education increase the demand for educated workers. When Bolles (1981) suggested that 80% of the population was underemployed, he was referring to the lack of full utilization of capabilities and the lack of challenge within work. This situation of underemployment may increase given advancing educational preparation and sophistication of workers who, especially in a tight fiscal milieu, remain at job levels and responsibilities below full capability.

There are those who suggest a shift in the centrality of work (Brown & Brooks, 1984). Work or careers are considered only a part of life, perhaps because they cannot meet all expectations nor be associated with feelings of self-worth to the extent that they have in the past. Career planning is being undertaken within a broader life perspective. Individuals seek options and satisfaction from a lifelong cycle that combines career with other life opportunities. Opportunities will be made for renewals at and away from work, such as time for sabbatical, self-study, play, and career-enrichment experiences. The fullest integration of the human potential movement in all aspects of one's life is receiving renewed emphasis.

Structure and Management of Work.   Increased competition, combined with studies of excellence in successful corporations (Peters & Waterman, 1982), bring new structures and management styles to the workplace. Bureaucracies are giving way to a new kind of democracy. Centralized, standardized, and top–down organizations that emphasized sameness and efficiency are giving way to decentralized approaches with priorities on innovation, entrepreneurship, and the "competitive edge." Some organizations are using matrix structures, grouping employees from various traditional departments around projects or special tasks. Other organizations are forming quality circles, and some foster participatory management. These successful organizations value unique and quality products as well as the personnel that make or define the new products or services.

Organizations striving for excellence want employees with career management skills. Persons with career perspectives and career management knowledge are becoming valued resources at an increasing rate. Organizations recognize that the employed person who has clear career goals more likely will be motivated toward quality performance and products. Also, persons managing their careers more often will be futurists, risk takers, effective negotiators, and transition makers. These skills and strategies, applied in a personal way to a career, can also be applied to an organization. Career managers, then, are sought and selected by current productivity-conscious, new-wave organizations that represent the organizational model for the future.

New and emerging structures in management of work are creating, if not demanding, new management and clinical advancement for nurses. Nurses, who are skilled in personal relationships, communication, and problem solving, can apply these skills to the management of health care agencies. The need for the clinically experienced person as product expert, manager, or administrator will become increasingly apparent in decentralized or honeycomb organizations. In addition, options will flourish as direct patient care, patient teaching, assistance with self-care, and a focus on mind/body integration become more obviously the prized products and outcome of the health care industry.

The Nature of the Workplace.   Workplaces increasingly are part of a multicorporate, diversified, and multinational conglomerate. Products or services emerge from multiservice and often international combinations of human, technologic, and natural resources. For example, the automotive industry combines raw steel from one country, technologic expertise from another, and human resources from yet another country. The combined product represents the best from many contributors.

We are witnessing similar changes in the health field. Many health agencies are part of very complex systems, including multi-hospital chains and multi-service corporations. For example, the Hospital Corporation of America (HCA), a large investor-owned hospital chain, owns and manages hospitals, skilled nursing facilities, and has interests in home care as well as hospital manufacturing and supply companies. Another corporation, American Medical International (AMI), operates acute care hospitals and respiratory treatment centers. Republic Health Corporation operates hospitals and mental health care facilities and manages substance abuse programs. Coleman (1984) predicts that eventually less than 100 "super systems" will control all the nation's health care. These super systems will amalgamate not only general hospitals and specialty hospitals, but diverse agencies such as home health services, long-term care facilities, minor emergency care services, surgery services, primary care centers, free-standing weight and fitness centers, health management services, and hospital supplies.

The changing nature of the workplace has tremendous implications for career management. The nurse in these complex systems will have greater opportunity for lateral mobility from acute to long-term or ambulatory care, from one clinical area to another, from one state to another, or even from nation to nation. Because the systems are more complex, sophisticated, and challenging, top- and middle-management positions will open up as well. With a goal, a plan, and effective networks and marketing skills, you will avoid feeling like a "small fish in a big sea" and capitalize on these burgeoning career opportunities.

Gender-Related Issues

The image of women and nurses as careerists is evolving. In the work force negative stereotypes gradually are giving way to the recognition that women with a career orientation are a formidable force, bringing unique skills in management, decision making, and communication. However, beliefs about women at work, socialization, stereotypes, and career barriers continue to influence many nurses in their careers.

Beliefs About Working Women. Misconceptions about both numbers and reasons for women working continue to exist. In fact, women comprise over one-half of all persons gainfully employed (Pinkstaff, 1979). Nurses, who number 1.6 million, represent a large percentage of that female work force. More than one-half of all adult women work, and more than two-thirds of women between 25 and 45 years old work (USNWR, 1984). Images often defy these facts, however. Approximately 75% of nurses who hold licenses work. Tenure is approximately 2.6 years in all industries and 2.7 years in the health industry. Hospital staff nurse turnover rates, although often believed to be high, are comparable to those of nonmanufacturing industries, which have an average turnover rate of about 24% annually (Institute of Medicine, 1983). Still, misconceptions exist about job retention and turnover rates among nurses.

Just as nurses work in greater numbers and as a more stable work force than commonly believed, they also work for different reasons. Consider your ideas about women working.

The belief that women work for extras, such as family vacations, a new refrigerator, or extra spending money, seems to persist despite the fact that most women work because of economic necessity. One in seven families is headed by a woman. Married women and the 57% of married women with children who work outside the home do so to maintain a moderate standard of living (USNWR, 1984). In addition to economic security, women seek and attain success, achievement, status, and a sense of fulfillment through their careers.

Common misconceptions such as ''Most women don't work,'' ''Women work to get out of the house,'' ''Women only work because they have to,'' or ''Women are not as stable at work because they have husbands to support them'' can influence your attitudes and others' perceptions about you as a member of the career world. Thus, it is exceedingly important for you to identify your own ideas about work and to assess the influence of any misconceptions on your nursing career.

Socialization. Development of gender role identity is an important influence in your career perspective. Children today, many of whom have working mothers and experience single-parent households, have a different gender-role socialization than in the past. Children now more than ever have an opportunity to see women as breadwinners who combine work with typical nurturing activities. With the women's movement, the concept of expanded gender roles is reinforced.

Today's working adults, however, are often influenced by early socialization. This can make careers in nursing difficult. From birth, many girls are still taught to give priority to nurturing roles and to reject competitive roles. Within the current health care environment, nurses may be slow to assert accomplishments, develop contacts, or realize the importance of competition. Nonassertive and noncompetitive behaviors can be contrary to management values and thwart nurses' autonomy and power within an organization. Perfectionism and overdevotion to service can also be counterproductive in the workplace, where a meshing of personal and organizational goals may be needed.

In nursing, men are often limited by gender role expectations. Unlike their female colleagues men in nursing are expected to be assertive, to deal with competition, and to seek positions of status and achievement. They may be expected to fill positions in emergency rooms, rehabilitation units, or operating rooms rather than in obstetric units, nurseries, or pediatric clinics. To what extent have you experienced the effects of gender role socialization on your nursing career?

Stereotypes. In the public's image, the media's portrayal of nursing, and among nurses themselves stereotypes abound. Most of these stereotypes have a basis in myth, yet are sprinkled with the realities of nursing's past. Stereotypes may have both positive and negative effects on nurses in their career management.

A common stereotype of the nurse is that of handmaiden. The public and physicians have viewed the nurse as one who follows orders. Nursing historically was performed by society's outcasts or by members of military and religious orders, and thus the image of humble obedience and submission to the control of others evolved.

Other common stereotypes, generally portrayed in novels, television dramatizations, pornographic movies, and greeting cards, are the nurse as sex symbol, sexpot, or battle-ax. As a counterpoint, the nurse with proper, clean, neat appearance and a starched cap represents the stereotype of the sweet, virginal girl in white. This is an attempt to place the nurse on a pedestal high above human, especially sexual, desires (Muff, 1982).

Another major bias is of nursing as an occupation that requires the characteristics of caring and nurturing, stereotypically female qualities. Medicine, on the other hand, is perceived with a diagnostic and treatment emphasis, qualities associated with the male sex. As a result, men in nursing are sometimes stereotyped as effeminate or as medical school dropouts. With more women entering medicine and more men entering nursing, and with nursing's language and practice encompassing diagnosis and treatment, these stereotypes will weaken.

Nursing leaders historically have been women, usually single, who are totally and solely committed to nursing. The dedicated nurse portrays this common stereotype. In the more recent past, nurses have rejected this image of total commitment, seeking a blend of nursing with other roles and responsibilities. The clearer dilineation of and emphasis on professional practice and client outcomes do much to focus the nurses' image on nursing. Have you experienced the effects of stereotypes on your career? Have they helped or hindered you? How do you see changing those stereotypes that limit you?

Barriers. Among the major barriers facing nurses are inequities in salary, limited access to executive level positions, and lack of support for child or home management.

Generally, women's salaries are approximately 62% of men's—a ratio that has remained constant for over 30 years (USNWR, 1984). This is partly because women are less skilled at the salary game. Also, many women are in service fields such as teaching, secretarial, and nursing, which perpetuates an overall lower income for women. Women and nurses in this decade face the issue of gaining equal pay for comparable work. Many cities in the United States have raised or are beginning to raise women's pay based on an analysis of job classifications and comparable worth evaluations. The economic effects of these decisions discourage broaching of similar comparable worth issues in private or nonprofit businesses, including health care agencies.

Between 1972 and 1981, nurses' salaries actually declined at an average rate of almost 1% per year (Institute of Medicine, 1983). In addition, nurses' salaries are not commensurate with their educational preparation or level of responsibility. Opportunities for change are evolving. Clinical and management ladders offer increased remunerative outcomes. Clinical nurse specialists, nurse researchers, executive nurse managers, and administrators are beginning to demand and be awarded more equitable salaries.

Hospitals, where the greatest numbers of nurses work, have male-dominated hierarchies that limit executive positions and maintain a fairly paternalistic relationship with nursing. Nurses without a department structure parallel to the medical model and without any influence on a board of directors have long experienced a diminished sense of autonomy and control over their own nursing practice within the hospital organization.

> The paternalism that keeps nurses subservient, underpaid, overworked, and personally and professionally fragmented from each other persists today. The trajectory of nursing's history cannot be challenged without an awareness of the impact of paternalism on nurses and nursing practice. Nurses can refuse to be wooed by paternal deception and exploitation. We must begin by shedding the fears and ignorance that make us amenable to external control. Our fears must be examined over and over again until they lose their power over us. Ignorance can be effectively decreased through reading, studying, and sharing our knowledge and experiences with other nurses. A united community of nurses actively sharing and working together to improve nursing practice will halt the abuses of paternalism and allow us to regain our personal and professional identities. (Lovell, 1982).

However, the competitive environment and changing structures in organizations are creating opportunities for women and nurses in particular. Decentralization in health care combined with the need to humanize the organization and its health services necessitate the placement of nurses in positions of managing and making policy decisions about health services and organizations.

Career barriers related to childbearing and family care remain important issues to nurses as they pursue their careers. The resulting guilt and anger associated with conflicts between work as a nurse and the demands of being a spouse, mother, and homemaker are strong and prevalent in the nursing work force. The burden of the "super nurse" or "super mom," trying to give equal time to all roles, can become intolerable, forcing choices between traditional homemaking and career roles. These choices may not be preferred but are resorted to when there is no exploration of work–life options. The expectation that child care, housework, and care of other dependent persons are typically feminine activities is gradually changing. Shared roles and guaranteed jobs after maternity or paternity leave will slowly become realities. The image of the nurse careerist racing, rushing, and trying to "do it all," saying "Isn't this what we are supposed to be able to do as full working professionals?" gradually is being replaced by the nurse who spaces, paces, and plans a career that blends with other life priorities.

Child and home care, salary, status, and power are barriers frequently experienced by nurses. Have you experienced any of these as barriers in your career? Surmounting them will be considerably easier if you anticipate and plan to diminish them through a career management process.

Exercise 1–1 Professional Concerns and Societal Issues

Consider your professional concerns and how societal changes influence them. The following questions may help you sift through relevant societal influences on selected nursing career concerns. After reading each question, briefly note in the spaces provided the relevant work and gender-related changes that may influence them.

1. Is it worth the time, effort, and money to get a doctorate in nursing so I can teach when the pay for teachers is less than the pay for staff nurses?

    Relevant issues: _____

    _____

    _____

2. As a self supporter with three children, which positions and strategies will insure that I can keep bread on the table?

    Relevant issues: _____

    _____

    _____

3. How can I achieve comparable pay and status in the hospital for doing the same, if not better, management than the non-nurse managers?

    Relevant issues: _____

    _____

    _____

4. What work and gender-related issues influence your career concerns? (Refer also to your questions on page 2.)

     _____

     _____

     _____

     _____

5. What societal issues influence your career concerns?

     _____

     _____

     _____

     _____

The purpose of this exercise is to help you validate or further appreciate the effects of societal changes such as work and gender-related issues on the nursing profession and on your career progression and management. The ability to identify and understand the direct and indirect effects of professional and societal changes on you and your career can also help you prevent or greatly diminish the effects of transitions and role stress.

Common Nursing Career Syndromes and Questions

With both the nursing profession and society in flux, nurses are prone to career problems. Career transitions and role stress are two of the most common syndromes.

Transitions

Transitions, or changes, from one role, setting, and culture to another characterize the work–lives of most people, especially nurses. Nurses experience many role transitions during their careers. RNs who return to school for higher degrees can anticipate the "return-to-school syndrome" (Shane, 1983). Graduates first entering the professional work force may experience "reality shock" (Kramer, 1974). The man or woman returning to work after time away from a career can experience problems in transition from home or school back to the work setting. Older nurses must integrate life losses (death of parents or spouses or the exit of children from the home) and anticipate professional retirement. Each work environment contains subcultures—administrative, professional, technical, and blue collar—that represent varying values and customs. Nurses make transitions to other cultural norms within many jobs and when changing jobs.

Phases of transition in roles, settings, and culture follow a pattern. There is an initial "honeymoon," with anticipation and excitement, followed by heightened conflict over disparities between the old and new, feelings of pressure to adjust, cope, or adapt, and ambivalence over the actual wisdom of the change. This conflict stage optimally is followed by resolution, when the best of the old is integrated with the new and the person is comfortable with the demands and values of both situations.

Transitions do not have to be times of crises. In transition you can learn new strategies for change and step forth with a stronger and clearer self-image to better assimilate new values, skills, and knowledge. In addition, use of career management strategies such as networking and attending to yourself become important to success. As more nurses return to school, then to work, and begin to influence both school and work cultures, more role models will be available to help guide the transitions.

Having a career goal in mind makes the struggles and adaptations during transitions seem worthwhile. A goal also allows you to effectively counter negative self-recriminations such as, "What am I doing in school with all these youngsters?" or "Why have I taken this position when all I do is worry about how my son is doing after school?" or "My friends all call me a bookworm." The negatives, whether from self or others, can be halted with the affirmation that "I really want to reach my career goal, and I'm on my way." A career plan helps with transitions because it involves planning measures to lessen conflict and strengthen supports.

Role Stress

Stress emerges from nursing roles that are ambiguous, contradictory, and unrealistic (Hardy, 1978). For instance, the role expectations for a clinical nurse specialist are vague in many organizations. Nonspecific duties, lack of clear delineation of accountability, and multiple reporting lines add to confusion about the role. Some roles carry contradictory messages such as those of a nurse supervisor who is expected to be an innovative and strong leader while maintaining the traditional feminine and deferential role. An example of unrealistic role expectations is the nurse clinician who is expected to be a primary nurse for a group of clients and simultaneously act as charge nurse in the absence of the unit coordinator.

Role stress evolves from unclear or overburdened roles, from conflict between personal values or skills and those that are expected for a role, and from changes in roles. Role stress, or more accurately distress, is evident when a person exhibits feelings of emotional helplessness or anger followed by mental confusion and narrow perception. If the stress continues, later symptoms include suspiciousness and altered self-image. Prolonged maladaptive anger is seen in passive–aggressive and obstructive negative responses (Smythe, 1984). The terminal phase of distress (inability to resolve work stress) is burnout.

Career management can help you prevent and treat role stress and burnout as well as shape answers to significant questions related to your career path.

Exercise 1–2   Where Are You?

Where are you today in your nursing career with regard to transitions and role stress? As you read the following possibilities, check any that apply to where you are today.

A. Are you at any of these turning points:

1. _____ In the last quarter/semester of your basic education program?

2. _____ A diploma or associate degree nursing graduate enrolled in a BSN program?

3. _____ Enrolled in a graduate program?

4. _____ In your first year of employment as a nurse?

5. _____ Seeking your first position as a nurse?

6. _____ Returning to work after being inactive in your nursing practice for two or more years?

7. _____ Approaching retirement?

B. Are you experiencing role stress because you are

8. _____ Considering expanding your role in nursing?

9. _____ Planning to change your position and/or level of responsibility?

10. _____ Moving from clinical practice to management responsibilities?

11. _____ Moving to a new work environment?

C. Are you experiencing feelings and frustrations that may be associated with role stress such as:

12. _____ Having trouble with your boss?

13. _____ Feeling overworked?

14. _____ Experiencing frustration because you are not asked to assume responsibilities that you want and are prepared to take?

15. _____ Feeling in conflict between professional and personal demands?

16. _____ Feeling that you are being asked to perform at a level above your current knowledge and skill?

17. _____ Feeling unsure and unclear about what is expected of you?

18. _____ Experiencing physical and emotional exhaustion related to your professional responsibilities?

19. _____ Feeling totally detached and uncaring about your performance?

20. _____ Experiencing frustration because you want to practice in the specific area of your expertise but are finding openings available only in your least-preferred clinical areas?

21. _____ Other? (Please write in) _____

_____

_____

_____

Knowing where you are in terms of a career transition and role stress can be a very enlightening step toward deciding where you want to be, what you want to do, and when you want to do it. Undertaking the process of career management will help you prevent or treat the negative effects of career transitions and role stress by instilling better understanding of the context in which they exist. Effective career management not only diminishes problems but promotes career vitality.

Attaining Career Vitality

Career vitality is an internal feeling of well-being, the sense that you are attaining what you want with your career. It is generated by optimal involvement and dedication to nursing practice and other activities related to your career in nursing. The nurse who is attaining career goals and experiencing career vitality usually enjoys work, believes that work makes a contribution to society, and sees a balance between rewards and efforts.

Nurses are seeking enjoyment from their work. They want to contribute and to feel as if their contribution to society is important. Nurses want to balance the practical rewards of status or money with the level of skills and knowledge invested in their nursing practice.

Enjoying Nursing

Enjoying nursing means experiencing success, productivity, and self-satisfaction from your involvement in nursing. The energy you invest in nursing is manifested through strong commitment and is rewarded by positive reinforcers compatible with your values, needs, and goals. Enjoying nursing allows you to cope with a multitude of stressors. Most of the time you view situations with confidence and openness to discern the range of possible meanings on which to base your actions. In the process of enjoying nursing, you perpetually encounter new experiences and constantly expand your knowledge. You acquire realistic expectations and the capacity for growth and change. You reach congruence between your ideal and your real self. You live dynamically in the present with the capacity for honest and realistic self-appraisal.

In the following case examples, Josie and Susan demonstrate their enjoyment of nursing with statements that indicate they experience success, productivity, and self-satisfaction from their involvement with the profession.

Case Example: Josie

Josie is a 24-year-old registered nurse who graduated from an associate degree nursing program 4 years ago. After working for 2 years on a general adult medical unit in her community, she enrolled in the university as a full-time student to complete her bachelor's degree in nursing. Josie's face beams when she says: "I really love nursing! I'm working nights and going to school full time too. I'm really excited about applying what I'm learning in school to my job and about my independent study this semester, where I'm having an opportunity to work with families and acutely ill children. I love teaching, and I have been offered a position teaching clinical nursing after I graduate."

Case Example: Susan

Susan is a clinical specialist on a maternity unit in a 200-bed community hospital. She is 36 years old and a wife and mother. "What I love about nursing," she states enthusiastically, "is working with patients at the bedside. This is something I think I do well, and I really enjoy it!"

Contributing to Society

Altruism, unselfish concern for the welfare of others, is historically associated with the image of nursing. The philosophies of schools of nursing include a common doctrine that the general welfare of society is the proper goal and responsibility of nursing. Belief in this doctrine gives essential purpose to nursing practice. The social significance of nursing contributes to its desirability as a career and to satisfaction with and pride in the profession. The belief that one makes a meaningful contribution to society is the hallmark of an effective nursing career and an essential ingredient of professional identity.

Styles' (1982) Declaration of Belief About the Nature and Purpose of Nursing states six beliefs about nursing:

1. I believe in nursing as an occupational force for social good, a
    force that, in the totality of its concern for all human health states

and for mankind's responses to health and environment, provides a distinct, unique, and vital perspective, value orientation, and service.

2. I believe in nursing as a professional discipline, requiring a sound education and research base grounded in its own science and in the variety of academic and professional disciplines with which it relates.

3. I believe in nursing as a clinical practice, employing particular physiological, psychosocial, physical, and technological means for human amelioration, sustenance, and comfort.

4. I believe in nursing as a humanistic field, in which the fullness, self-respect, self-determination, and humanity of the nurse engage the fullness, self-respect, self-determination, and humanity of the client.

5. I believe that nursing's maximum contribution for social betterment is dependent on: (a) The well-developed expertise of the nurse; (b) The understanding, appreciation and acknowledgement of that expertise by the public; (c) The organizational, legal, economic, and political arrangements that enable the full and proper expression of nursing values and expertise; (d) The ability of the profession to maintain unity within diversity.

6. I believe in myself and in my nursing colleagues: (a) In our responsibilities to develop and dedicate our minds, bodies, and souls to the profession that we esteem and the people whom we serve; (b) In our right to be fulfilled, to be recognized, and to be rewarded as highly valued members of society.

These beliefs sensitively applied to self, to others, and to nursing strike an essential balance between altruism, humanism, and self-advocacy, which empowers nurses in their quest for harmony between professionhood and selfhood and the healthy integration of self and career.

Balance Between Rewards and Efforts

A balance between rewards and efforts is important for career satisfaction. Rewards are both intrinsic and extrinsic. Intrinsic rewards are individual psychologic satisfiers such as a sense of accomplishment and belonging and being valued for your significant contribution to the organization. Examples of extrinsic rewards include remuneration in proportion to responsibilities; sufficient medical, vacation, and other benefits; and a pleasant work environment.

Because of the social significance of nursing, intrinsic rewards usually outweigh extrinsic rewards. Thanks to collective bargaining, nurses' salaries and benefits have improved in many geographic regions. Intrinsic rewards continue to play a key role in career satisfaction for nurses. Awareness of both kinds of rewards is important to effectively managing your own career.

Exercise 1–3   Career Vitality

Considering where you are in your nursing career, reflect on your enjoyment of nursing, your beliefs about its importance, and the balance of rewards with your efforts. Write your reflections in the space provided.

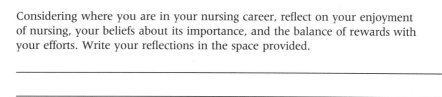

Your personal reflections on career vitality start you toward the optimal management of your career in nursing. In this chapter you have explored issues and experiences that verify the relevance and importance of career management. This is the first of several phases of a personal and professional process for managing your career in nursing. In Chapter 2 you will have the opportunity to explore and enhance your career management perspective further.

References

ANA delegates vote to limit RN title to BSN grad; Associate nurse wins vote for technical title. *AJN* 1985; *85:* 1016–1022.

Bolles R: *What Color is Your Parachute?* Berkeley, CA: Ten Speed Press, 1981.

Brown D et al: *Career choice and Development,* p. 408. San Francisco, CA: Jossey-Bass, 1984.

Coleman J, Dayani E, Simms E: Nursing careers in the emerging systems. *Nurs Management* 15(1): 23, 1984.

Hardy M. Role stress and role strain. In: *Role Theory: Perspectives for Health Professionals,* pp. 73–109. Hardy ME, Conway M (editors). New York: Appleton-Century-Crofts, 1978.

Institute of Medicine: *Nursing and Nursing Education: Public Policies and Private Actions,* pp. 192–193; 197. Washington, DC: National Academy Press, 1983.

Kramer M: *Reality Shock: Why Nurses Leave Nursing.* St. Louis: Mosby, 1974.

Lovell M: Daddy's little girl: The lethal effects of paternalism in nursing. In: *Socialization, Sexism and Stereotyping*, p. 210. Muff J. (editor). St. Louis: Mosby, 1982.

Muff J (editor): *Socialization, Sexism and Stereotyping*, p. 127. St. Louis: Mosby, 1982.

Nursing: A Social Policy Statement. Kansas City, MO: American Nurses' Association, 1980.

Peters TJ, Waterman R: *In Search of Excellence.* New York: Harper & Row, 1982.

Pinkstaff M, Wilkinson A: *Women at Work: Overcoming the Obstacles*, p. 17. Menlo Park, CA: Addison-Wesley, 1979.

Shane D: *Returning to School.* Englewood Cliffs, NJ: Prentice-Hall, 1983.

Smythe E: *Surviving Nursing*, pp. 38–57. Menlo Park, CA: Addison-Wesley Publishing Company, 1984.

Styles M: *On Nursing: Toward a New Endowment, p. 61.* St. Louis: Mosby, 1982.

Ten forces reshaping America. *USNWR* 1984; 96(11):47.

2 A Career Perspective

FRANCES C. HENDERSON
BARBARA O. McGETTIGAN

Managing your career so that you reach realistic career goals requires a certain perspective about nursing—a career perspective. This perspective enables you to view nursing not as just a job but as one integral part of life and a work–life whole. As a career, nursing is a *personal* experience, a *developmental* process, and a *self-directed* pursuit.

A nursing career is very personal because it expresses your personality and serves as a means of meeting needs and attaining individual fulfillment. As a developmental process, your career in nursing continuously advances over the life span not necessarily in the sense of you moving up the ladder, but in the sense of you achieving fuller and richer self-realization. Your career requires and allows development of increasingly complex skills to accomplish increasingly complex tasks and demands ever-deepening reflections over your lifetime.

To gain a comprehensive career perspective, take time to explore how a job and career differ; analyze the part career plays in your life; and review the needs, stage, and degree of self-direction within your nursing career.

Beyond a Job

The line between job and career represents an orientation to what you are doing. With a job orientation, you perform assigned, discrete tasks and fulfill responsibilities as established in a job description. You depend on your boss for opportunities, rewards, and benefits. You accept a job, and formally or informally contract to meet the requirements established by the employer.

Table 2–1   Job and Career Differences

Job definition	Career definition
A position that is accepted	A chosen path
A contract made with an employer to meet position requirements	A contract made with yourself, based on your career plan, to fulfill personal and professional goals
A set of discrete tasks performed according to a job description	A pattern and sequence of positions and activities that move you toward your career goal
Day-to-day employment	Satisfying employment for now and the future

Unlike a job, which is directed by someone else, a *career* is a pursuit that you design and promote. With a career orientation, you strive to use a flexible repertoire of skills and to act on your key life values. Rather than performing tasks, you focus on goals and purpose. Your purpose essentially is a contract with yourself to realize personal and professional goals and to reap the satisfaction of self-fulfillment. As a career-oriented person you may combine jobs or move from agency to agency or job to job, building a career on various positions. Your career moves form a sequence, a pattern that reflects you, your goals, and your plan. Not limited by a day-to-day focus, you are directed to the future.

Refer to Table 2–1. Contrast the phrases and adjectives for job and career. Is nursing a job or a career for you?

Most of us seek more than a job. As one worker, interviewed by Terkel (1975), said, "I think most of us are looking for a calling, not a job. Most of us . . . have jobs that are too small for our spirit. Jobs are not big enough for people." These comments express the common human goal of seeking opportunities that acknowledge the fullness of our being. Whether within our career, our family, or community work, we strive to actualize ourselves.

A Part of a Work–Life Whole

The emphasis and amount of energy or work expended on a career varies from person to person, and, for any one person, at different times of life. Other aspects of your life to which you channel energy or work and enact roles include home and family, education, personal development, leisure, health, and community. Together with your career, all aspects of your life comprise a work–life whole.

Work–life whole is a term conveying the unity of life that emerges as various roles are enacted and tasks are undertaken in concert with each other. Each person assumes numerous roles, combining, for example, family and career at one point in life and perhaps adding the leisure role at another time. As roles change, the complexity and demands of the tasks involved also change. The tasks within a role, from exploring and establishing, to maintaining and flourishing, to final diminishing effort, have a natural pattern applied in unique ways by persons in various roles. For instance, a person might be exploring a career, establishing a homemaker role, but declining emphasis on being a student as graduation becomes imminent. This interplay between roles and tasks creates a very personal life–career kaleidoscope (Super, 1984) or work–life whole.

Figure 2–1 illustrates a work–life whole in which an individual devotes the same amount of energy toward each of six components. This balance is rarely, if ever, the case. The importance of career shifts as individuals move through the life span and other life aspects demand priority. For example, Figure 2–2 reflects an individual's emphasis on family. This could represent a woman in early adulthood raising a young infant. It could also refer to an adult caring for an aging parent during middle adulthood, or an elderly person spending precious energy and time rediscovering the joys and mimicry of his or her grandchildren's play. In each example, family is the major life focus with a concurrent de-emphasis on career. Figure 2–3 shows equal emphasis on career and community. The person depicted here might be an older adult adjusting to retirement and simultaneously volunteering services. This could also represent a middle-aged woman who is active politically and at the same time re-establishing herself in a profession after a career interruption. Thus, a

Figure 2–1   Example of a work–life whole with equal emphasis on six components.

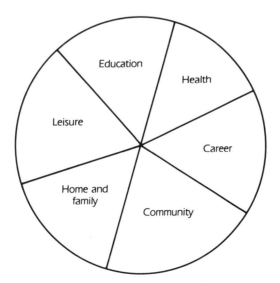

Figure 2–2 Example of a work–life whole showing emphasis on the family.

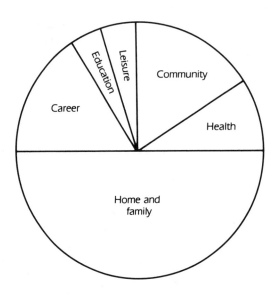

Figure 2–3 Example of a work–life whole showing equal emphasis on career and community.

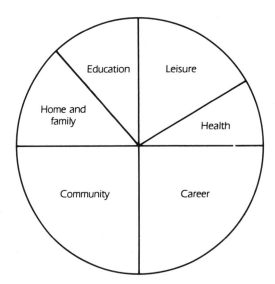

great deal of fluctuation often occurs in the importance or emphasis that a person places on a career from early, through middle, to later adulthood.

Despite the traditional view that a career is most important during early and middle adulthood, it can be as or more important for some in late adolescence or late adulthood. Also, career emphasis fluctuates during the life span, consuming time for some years, then receding in importance as different life aspects come to the forefront.

Your career interacts to support, supplement, complement, or conflict with the other aspects of a work–life whole. In one situation career advancement may cause stress, affecting health and limiting community or family involvement. In another situation advancement of a career may foster such self-realization that involvement in the family or community flourishes. A thriving family life can support efforts needed to change or reenter a nursing career, whereas establishing a new family can divert energies from career advancement. Awareness of this interrelationship of career and other life aspects leads you to appreciate, anticipate, and plan for the effects of changes in career and other life roles and tasks. Your career goals and plans are made and managed most effectively in relation to a broad life plan, a work–life whole.

Exercise 2–1   Profiles of Your Work–Life Whole

Consider your present work–life whole. Using the circle provided here, create segments that represent the amount of time and energy you now devote to the six aspects of life: leisure, community, career, home and family, health, education or personal development. Your circle should look like a pie that you have sliced into various-sized pieces. You may want to add shading to indicate the intensity or complexity of the tasks involved in each of your life roles.

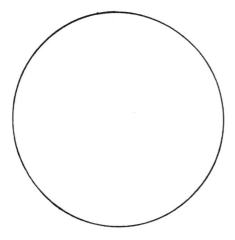

Now that you have drawn your profile, reflect on whether this has changed over the last 5 years. What can you anticipate about changes in the next 5 years? Create a profile in the following circle that depicts your anticipated allocation of time and priorities in 5 years.

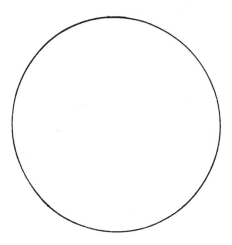

A Personal Experience

Your nursing career fulfills needs and portrays who you are in a very unique and personal way. Depending on your level of need, nursing may satisfy basic security needs or provide a means for full expression of your capabilities.

Figure 2–4 is an adaptation of Hagberg and Leider's (1978) representation of Maslow's Hierarchy of Needs related to careers. It illustrates that a person who predominantly meets security needs for food and shelter is more often job focused. Satisfying ego needs of recognition, esteem, or status through career pursuits becomes possible after the basic needs are met. For instance, a newly divorced single parent might focus only on meeting basic needs through a job. A person who has lived through an economic depression might vigilantly insure that work brings security by focusing on basic needs. Conversely, a person who has never experienced financial insecurities or who has attained a level of economic security may strive for social status or personal esteem from a career.

Based on the needs and realities of life at any given time, you function at various levels as you move toward self-actualization in your career. You experience the most complete satisfaction from your career when your work enables you to express fully and develop the capabilities, characteristics, style, and person that you are.

Consider your present involvement in nursing, keeping in mind your

Figure 2–4   Needs related to career.

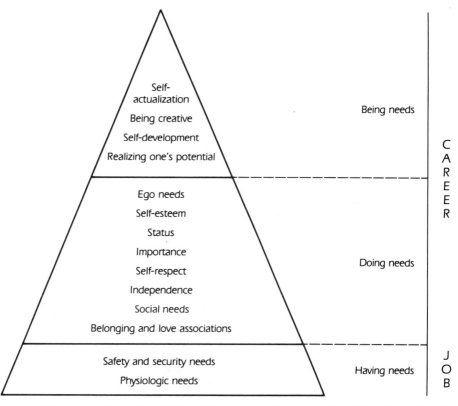

Adapted with permission from Hagberg J, Leider R: *The Inventurers: Excursions in Life and Career Renewal*, p. 87. Reading, MA: Addison-Wesley, 1978.

work–life whole. If your time and energies are deployed in other work–life areas, you may be actualizing your potential in areas other than your nursing career. At this phase in your life, what needs does nursing fulfill? Is nursing meeting basic needs or is it satisfying higher level needs?

Exercise 2–2   Career and Needs

A. Think of the roles and activities associated with your work as a nurse. Place a check mark next to the following statements that apply to you.
My nursing work is currently:

1. _____   An activity by which I earn a living

2. _____   An activity by which I build my self-esteem

3. _____ An opportunity to interact meaningfully with others

4. _____ An opportunity to grow both personally and professionally

5. _____ A central theme of my life

6. _____ An opportunity to gain status

7. _____ A way to fulfill my obligation to work for a living

8. _____ A way to express my skills and talents

9. _____ A means of providing for my retirement

10. _____ Other (please write in) _____

_____

B. Assess your findings from the statements you checked.

1. What is the highest level of need that your work in nursing meets? Place a check mark next to one of the following levels.

_____ Having needs (If you checked 1, 7, 9, or wrote in others that are similar)

_____ Doing needs (If you checked 2, 3, 6, or wrote in others that are similar)

_____ Being needs (If you checked 4, 5, 8, or wrote in others that are similar)

2. Are you satisfied with the level of need that nursing now meets for you? Are there other needs you want to meet through your work in nursing? Make a note here of what you want from your nursing career.

_____

_____

_____

In addition to meeting personal needs, your nursing career is a portrait of you. It expresses many dimensions, such as your personality characteristics, attributes, style, and stage. Your career goals, plan, and the application of career strategies emerge from and convey your many dimensions. *Personality characteristics* include your needs, values, and interests. *Attributes* refer to both skills attained and subjects you are knowledgeable in from your work in nursing, school, leisure, or elsewhere. Other dimensions are your style and stage. *Style* is evident in your approach to life in general and to people and selected tasks. *Stage* represents your place along the mental, physical, psychosocial, and developmental continuum, and your level of professional expertise.

The career goals you establish evolve from a consideration of what you value, your interests, preferences, as well as needs. Your personal values direct your beliefs about work and the organizations, roles, and activities associated with your career. Without this personal awareness and portrayal, your career goals are empty and have little chance of promoting satisfaction or actualization of your potential as a nurse. For instance, if you are a very private and investigative person, a career goal of laboratory research will mean more than a goal of becoming an organizational leader.

Career plans also derive from considering specific actions and time frames that will work for you. The career strategies you use must suit you. For instance, belonging to an association may be effective networking for one person, but another may find a small group of peers more appropriate to personal style and level of experience.

Self-awareness is therefore basic to effective career choice. Self-awareness means paying attention and being open to yourself. Appreciate your inner workings as you appreciate the beating of your heart. Admit to yourself and others how important your characteristics are. Don't judge how you "measure up" to an external yardstick or describe how you could or should be. Acknowledge what is true for yourself, using an internal reality as the standard. Whether positive or negative, strength or weakness, success or failure, charm or foible, personality characteristics, traits, and style must be recognized, appreciated, and accepted as your "reasonable boundaries" (Smythe, 1984).

In many cases we are our own worst critics, unwilling to accept our personal strengths. Think for a moment of a situation where you were complimented for a job well done but felt that you could have done better. Perfectionists and high achievers experience these feelings most often. As learners, adults also commonly underestimate their knowledge, performance, and potential. For example, how many times were you surprised with a high score on a written test? Difficulties and shortcomings of testing tools aside, adults often are unaware or unaccepting of the amount of information gained through experience or education. Is your appraisal of your knowledge, performance, and potential realistic? If asked, what would you say you do well? Are you aware of your knowledge and skills but unaware of other personal dimensions such as values, interests, and style? Consider your degree of self-awareness by completing Exercise 2–3.

Exercise 2–3   Degree of Self-Awareness

Rank the following personal dimensions on a scale from 1 to 4, according to degree of self-awareness (1, no awareness; 2, minimal awareness; 3, attuned or aware; 4, acknowledge and verbalize awareness). Circle the number that reflects your degree of awareness for each dimension.

	Degree of awareness			
Personal dimensions				
Personality characteristics	None	Minimal	Aware	Aware and verbalize
Needs	1	2	3	4
Values	1	2	3	4
Interests	1	2	3	4
Attributes				
Skill preference	1	2	3	4
Special knowledge	1	2	3	4
Style				
Lifestyle	1	2	3	4
Learning style	1	2	3	4
Communication style	1	2	3	4
Stage				
Psychosocial stage	1	2	3	4
Professional skill level and experience	1	2	3	4

Scoring

Use the following steps to obtain your total score.

Step 1: Add the numbers circled in each column to obtain your subtotals: _____ + _____ + _____ + _____

Step 2: Add the subtotals to obtain your total score: _____ + _____ + _____ + _____ = _____

Interpretation. A maximally aware person, one who acknowledges and verbalizes self-awareness in all dimensions, would have a total score of 40. If you scored below 30 you need to work on tuning in to your own personal thoughts and feelings. (Chapter 5 provides specific tools and exercises to assist you in recognizing or confirming your personality characteristics, attributes, style, and stage.)

Think of yourself in relation to your career as an artist doing a self-portrait. The artist makes a profile by combining internal perceptions of how he or she looks with the actual image he or she sees. Colors are chosen, according to intensity and tone, which can convey feelings, connote ideas, or create a mood of the artist. Depending on his or her particular school or approach, the artist may copy a mirror reflection precisely and realistically, apply a more interpretive or impressionistic approach, or even make a caricature. Like the artist, we all express ourselves in a career in different ways, according to individual backgrounds and emphasis. The unique results represent the needs and personality of each of us.

A Developmental Process

The course a career takes forms a pattern. Career patterns emerge as a series of developmental tasks, or stages, that you undertake during your life and as the way you think about and understand your career.

Career Stage

As a nurse, you assess many aspects of human development: physical, psychologic, intellectual, and moral. You assess a client's physical development and place it along the continuum of normal aging. You also recognize the level and appropriateness of psychologic tasks such as degree of intimacy for an adolescent or trust for an infant. A person experiences career development similar to the physical or psychological dimensions of growth and development. Career development involves gaining sophistication with increasingly complex career tasks at various stages of your life.

Central goals or themes related to career are reflected in life stages from childhood through older adulthood. In very early childhood, play is the means of learning about work and work roles. The pre-schooler often is seen literally wearing the shoes of others, play-acting the various roles of working adults. Further development of interests and capabilities needed for career decision making and for learning about various jobs occurs in the middle years of childhood. Adolescents develop tentative job interests and values and consider more specific work opportunities either in fantasy or in summer or after-school jobs.

Adult developmental tasks related to careers have been charted with varying time spans and labels by many authors and researchers. For example, Sheehy (1976) refers to the "Trying Twenties, Catch Thirties, Forties Crucible, and Final Renewal." Super (1969) describes the "trial explorations" of the 17 to 24-year-old person, the "establishment" stage of the 24 to 44-year-old person, the "maintenance" work of the 44 to 64-year-old person, and the "deceleration" of the 64 to 70-year-old person. Levinson (1978) describes a similar pattern, delineating 10-year phases, with roughly 6 years of stability followed by 4 years of transition to and from each stable phase. Levinson states that a person generally leaves family to establish work between the ages of 20 and 29 years. Between 30 and 40 years of age, a person settles down but may experience a midlife transition, attempting to reach out and fully express other aspects of the self. A period of restabilization between ages 40 and 45 is followed by full career and life realization at age 50. The older adult makes a transition toward retirement.

Table 2–2   Adult Developmental Stages

Age	Phase	Central purposes and pervasive themes	Your benchmark
18–22	Transition to adulthood	Exploring intimacy, independence, identity, involvement, and ideals; wondering what you should do	
23–30	Young adulthood	Experiencing involvement with intimates, self-sufficiency, self-identity, and commitment to ideals; doing what you should do	
30–37	Adulthood	Assuming responsibility for intimacy, identity, involvement, and ideals; juggling roles and responsibilities; knowing what you should do, wondering if you can	
38–45	Transition to mid-adulthood	Reviewing and revising previous decisions; openness to alternatives; exerting and asserting yourself; thinking what you can do, and doing it	
46–53	Mid-adulthood	Balancing your life; renewed stability and vitality; enjoying self-confidence and security; doing what you know you can do	
54–61	Transition to later adulthood	Changing your sense of self and others; integrating yourself with your life choices; being, doing, and enjoying it	
62–69	Later adulthood	Exploring alternatives; viewing life horizons; modeling ideals and values; doing what you like and liking what you do	
70–	Senior adulthood	Self approval; doing what you are able; remembering what you did	

Table 2–2 is an adaptation from several career theorists (Super, 1969, 1984; Sheehy, 1976; Levinson et al, 1978). It offers some central purposes and pervasive themes of careers at various stages in the adult years.

Exercise 2– 4   A Personal Review of Career Stage and Tasks

Review Table 2–2. Identify the central purposes and pervasive themes that pertain to you at this point in your life. In the column provided place a check next to your present place along the developmental continuum. You may be within a stage or between stages. Your position is your benchmark, from which you anticipate and note future changes. It allows you to appreciate more completely your total life pattern and its natural sequence.

In the space provided here, write your thoughts about reviewing career stages. Note consistencies or inconsistencies between central purposes and themes and your age.

1.   Reviewing career stages made me think that _____

_____

_____

_____

2.   The consistency between my career stage and age is _____

_____

For me that means _____

_____

This review of career stages probably confirms that your career is not just for you now, this year, or next year; it is lifelong. You will continue to develop as a career person as long as you continue to make decisions about your career and plan and manage your life work. Reviewing career stages also illustrates the overriding order, the natural ebb and flow, of your career life, which can help you understand, anticipate, and cope with the seemingly endless transitions from one stage to another. Finally, exploring career stages highlights the increasing complexity of the decision-making tasks you must undertake with your career throughout your career life.

Be cautious when applying concepts of career stages in your life. Career stages merely describe tasks over time and cannot reflect the unique meaning of your own tasks or time frames. For example, you may deal with central goals or undertake career tasks of one stage for a longer or shorter period than shown in Table 2–2. Your pace makes your developmental sequence unique. Stages may overlap or you may experience stages not associated with chronologic age. Life events rather than chronologic age often influence adult career development. A delay or re-entry into a career, a retirement, or an involuntary shift to an entirely new career due to poor health or economics will sequence and pace your career stages in a way that is your own.

The experience of being "out of sync" compared to the typical tasks of others may cause frustration or feelings that your career is going against a natural course. On the other hand, proceeding at a different pace may bring you a sense of prestige or advantage. Keep in mind that you evolve uniquely toward career fulfillment and actualization. What matters is that maturity toward career satisfaction does occur. This internal development is what is important, not keeping time with an external clock devised by others, competing, or comparing yourself with others.

Ideas About Career

You also develop in the way you think about a career and in your level of understanding what a career is. Knefelkamp and Slepitza (1976; 1978) describe a series of stages in thinking about career that progresses from a stage of dualistic thinking, through stages of multiplicity and relativism, and finally to a stage of commitment within relativism. In studying students at different ages,

Knefelkamp and others found key differences in what they say over time about their careers and how they describe a career. For instance, Valiga (1982) finds that most senior nursing students reflect a dualistic way of thinking about their careers. In this phase, a person views a career with a right-or-wrong, black-or-white, either-or, absolutist orientation. Statements that reflect this absolutist thinking include: "I will choose this service career because I hate business options," or "I must be certain that this is the right direction."

In the next phase of development, multiplicity, a person emphasizes exploring or analyzing many options, seeking and gathering multiple or varied ideas, but following the "right" steps of the decision-making process to the letter. A person in this phase uses fewer absolutes in talking about a career and is more introspective about personal strengths, weaknesses, and traits. The idea persists, however, that the right answers will be found if only enough exploration and problem solving are done. Typical comments might be: "I am so confused because I have so many things to consider such as skill and interests," or "I need to search and understand everything that's out there."

Individuals in the next stage, relativism, usually want to understand the variety of options, explore the positive and negative aspects of each, and visualize themselves in a variety of roles. A person in this stage is not looking for the one best direction but realizes that several career pathways may be more or less satisfying. There is an ability to take responsibility, to make a career plan, and to implement that plan. In the stage of relativism a certain amount of mourning occurs for all the options that will no longer be possible when a specific direction is taken. The person shows a certain reluctance to take control and plunge ahead for fear of what will be missed. Typical statements that reflect this stage of relativist thinking about a career are: "I really want to be very open and flexible and have a variety of things to do," or "I've weighed the advantages and disadvantages of each alternative, and the best for me at this time is this."

The last stage in developing a concept about a career is referred to as commitment. Interestingly, in a study of 100 generic nursing students, Collins (1981) found no baccalaureate nursing student who had achieved a level of commitment. Even at a doctoral level students often have not attained commitment. At this stage, a person has dealt with the variety of alternatives and made a synthesis between career and self. There is a commitment to specific career objectives and a clear direction, similar to a mission. There is an excellent match between self and career. A person with career commitment has a direction that constantly unfolds and provides for full devotion and use of career energy. With this stance, a person is willing to take risks or expand current roles with awareness, confidence, and satisfaction because career directions are clear, strong, and come from within. Statements that express a career at the commitment stage include: "What I am about is my work with media in preventive health," or "My personal themes really are being expressed through my work as a part-time hospice volunteer and parent."

Figure 2–5   Adaptation of the model of career development variables of qualitative change. Degree of density corresponds with presence of variable.

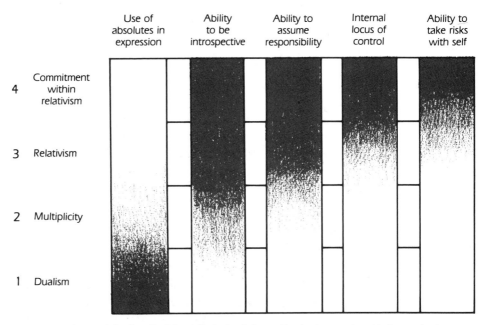

Adapted with permission from Knefelkamp LL, Slepitza R: A cognitive developmental model of career development—an adaptation of the Perry scheme. *Counseling Psychol* 1976; 6(3):53–58.

Exercise 2–5   Assessing Your Career Development

Review Figure 2–5. Rank the defining variables or characteristics described here on a scale from 1 to 4, according to the extent you believe each typifies you (1, most typical; 2, usually typical; 3, somewhat typical; 4, not typical). Circle the number that reflects how typical these behaviors are for you.

Defining Behaviors	Very typical	Usually typical	Somewhat typical	Not typical
a. I use a lot of absolutes—right-or-wrong statements—when I describe my career.	1	2	3	4
b. I avoid looking inward to assess my traits, strengths, or weaknesses; I am not introspective.	1	2	3	4
c. I avoid developing a career plan.	1	2	3	4
d. I rely on my supervisor or peers to advise me about what to do with my career.	1	2	3	4

Defining Behaviors	Very typical	Usually typical	Somewhat typical	Not typical
e. I shun different positions or new tasks at work.	1	2	3	4
f. I am not interested in seeing how well new tasks seem to fit me.	1	2	3	4

Scoring

Obtain your score by following the given steps.

Step 1: Add the numbers circled in each column.

Step 2: Total them: _____ + _____ + _____ + _____

Step 3: Divide the sum by 6 to obtain your score: _____ ÷ 6 = _____

Transfer your score to the stage on Figure 2–5: 1 = dualism; 2 = multiplicity; 3 = relativism; 4 = commitment within relativism.

Interpretation. Your behaviors may give you clues to your stage of career development. Through internal and progressive steps—from thinking and feeling that there is only one career direction to a gradual understanding of many possible options—a career direction is chosen and cherished because it expresses who you are in your career.

A Self-Directed Pursuit

A career does not just happen; it is actively engineered. The key element is you—active and self-directed—choosing your path, designing your plan, and guiding the course of your actions. Being self-directed means you believe in yourself and in your ability to make things happen. You don't have a "what will be will be" attitude, but feel you can change what might happen tomorrow by what you do today. Most of the time you try hard because you know you can influence the outcome. You resist the attitude that "problems are solved if you leave them alone" and actively seek solutions and plan ahead. You realize that you make your own opportunities by honing your talents and cultivating contacts. You recognize that real opportunity depends on your readiness to meet personal goals and your willingness to take risks. In addition, you believe you can create your own opportunities, not just wait for the right circumstances.

Self-direction in your career can be compared to being a master surfer. Picture yourself trying to ride the crest of a wave. You know your own style and your strong points; you know the surf and how to read the breaking of the waves; you have learned strategies for getting into the wave at just the right time. If the timing isn't right for the wave coming up behind you, you try the next good wave. You may tumble, but you will not be thrown entirely. You know the ocean is unpredictable, but you have a sense of its rhythm. You know yourself and you are in charge. You enjoy the challenge of the surf. You have your sights on shore and know about where you will surface. You know that the biggest waves take you where the rocks and risky terrain lie, but you experience such joy and gratification riding the waves along that way to shore.

Being self-directed in your career means you plan the moves along your path. At the same time, you recognize that life is not stable and requires constant reconsideration and adaptation. Through the process of planning and managing your career, you reap the joys of riding your own wave of career destiny.

Self-direction becomes a stronger and deeper quality over time. Also, you may feel more or less self-directed at different points in your life. When you have experienced a personal crisis such as a divorce or death of a spouse, you may rely on others' recommendations for a time, but you will regain career control as your personal life stabilizes.

Generally, decisions about careers both mirror and are influenced by personal ego development (Knefelkamp et al, 1978; Tiedeman & Miller-Tiedeman, 1984). At earlier stages in personal development we act impulsively and at later, more mature levels, we analyze decisions with a respect for self within the context of others' rights and responsibilities. In a similar fashion career decision making follows a sequence from impulsiveness and little or no direction, to being influenced by others, and then to full self-direction. Refer to Table 2–3, which lists the levels of developing self-direction in your career and

Table 2–3   Toward Developing Self-Direction

Level	Description	Definition
Without direction	Career is a reaction	Person acts impulsively and without goals; depends on others, feels aimless
	Career is on hold	Person is afraid to move forward; is self-protective, feels stymied
Other-directed	Career is a response	Person complies or conforms to others and wants to gain or maintain others' approval; feels helpless, out of control
Self-directed	Career is planned	Self-aware person assumes responsibility for what happens Conscientiously establishes methods to achieve personal purpose; feels in charge, in control
	Career is a synthesis	Person tailors plans to integrate self with roles and responsibilities to others and society; acts autonomously and cherishes individuality Feels exuberance, satisfaction, and commitment; career is integrated into total life

describes how each level feels. To consider the degree of self-direction reflected in your choice to pursue nursing, complete Exercise 2–6.

Exercise 2–6 Influences on Your Choice of Nursing

Given the following statements, check those that influenced your initial decision to choose nursing as a career.

1. A career in nursing is something I always wanted.

2. A career in nursing was one of a limited number of career choices acceptable to my family.

3. Pursuing a nursing career was something I could afford at the time.

4. A career in nursing is something my significant other always wanted for me.

5. Nursing was one of the career choices that interested me.

6. A career in nursing was a quick means to gain a position by which I could support or help support my family.

7. I was advised by a counselor to pursue a career in nursing.

8. I pursued a nursing career because there was an opening in the school.

9. I pursued a nursing career because it was what my best friend was doing.

Interpretation.   You may note the differences in the character of these statements. Items 1, 3, 5, and 6 are statements that connote self-direction. These indicate that you chose to pursue nursing for your own reasons such as stable employment, interest, or desire. These or other internal reasons may continue to influence your current pursuit of nursing. If you checked statements 2, 4, or 7, your initial choice of nursing was influenced by others. For instance, responding to a counselor or to family expectations placed the center of control with others and away from yourself. Going along with whatever was happening with friends or circumstances (statements 8 and 9) reflects a reactive mode in your initial choice of a nursing career.

Your entry into nursing may have stemmed from your internal direction or from external forces and circumstances. Consider where you are now with self-direction in your career. Are you working from day to day without a conscious career goal? Do you feel somewhat aimless? Are you continuing to live out someone else's dream or expectations? To attain a full career in nursing, you need to free yourself from living out messages of others from the past. You need to claim nursing as your personal choice and establish personal goals and plans. Reaching career goals and attaining a personal expression and fulfillment from a career evolve from affirmation of that career choice as what you want. It involves assuming direction of your own career pursuit.

In this chapter you have reviewed what your career means to you. Perhaps you now more fully appreciate or more laudably validate that your career is a very personal, developmental, and self-directed aspect of your life. The next chapter provides a framework and method for career management, enabling you to turn your desires into action.

References

Collins MS: *An investigation of the development of professional commitment in baccalaureate nursing students,* doctoral dissertation. Syracuse University, New York. *Dissert Abstr* 1981; 42: 1820 B.

Hagberg J, Leider R: *The Inventurers: Excursions in Life and Career Renewal,* p. 87. Menlo Park, CA: Addison-Wesley, 1978.

Knefelkamp L et al: Jane Loevinger's milestones of development. In: *Applying New Developmental Findings.* L Knefelkamp et al (editors). No. 4: *New Directions for Student Services,* pp. 69–91. San Francisco: Jossey-Bass, 1978.

Knefelkamp L, Slepitza R: A cognitive developmental model of career development—An adaptation of the Perry scheme. *Counseling Psychol* 1976; 6 (3): 53–58.

Knefelkamp L, Slepitza R:. A cognitive developmental model of career development—A relook at its descriptive stages. University of Maryland, College Park, 1978. Available from Perry Development Scheme Network c/o Larry Copes, ISEM, 10429 Barnes Way, St. Paul, MN 55075.

Levinson D et al: *The Seasons of a Man's Life.* New York: Knopf, 1978.

Sheehy G: *Passages: Predictable Crises of Adult Life.* New York: Bantam, 1976.

Smythe E: *Surviving Nursing,* p. 61. Menlo Park, CA: Addison-Wesley, 1984.

Super DE: Natural history of a study of lives and vocations. *Perspect on Educ* 1969; 2: 13–22.

Super DE: Career life development. In: *Career Choice and Development,* pp. 192–234. Brown D, Brooks L (editors). San Francisco: Jossey-Bass, 1984.

Terkel S: *Working,* p. XXIX. New York: Avon, 1975.

Tiedeman D, Miller-Tiedeman A: Career decision making: An individualistic process. In: *Career choice and development,* p. 308. Brown D, Brooks L (editors). San Francisco: Jossey-Bass, 1984.

Valiga T: *The cognitive development and perception about nursing as a profession of baccalaureate nursing students,* doctoral dissertation. Teacher's College, Columbia University, New York. *Dissert Abstr* 1982; 43 (5): 1447 A.

3 Framework of Career Management for Nurses

BARBARA O. McGETTIGAN
FRANCES C. HENDERSON

The framework of career management for nurses is a multifaceted structure that identifies key components and processes for establishing and validating a specific career path. How the components and processes of the framework interrelate forms a design for career management for nurses. The framework is based on the philosophy that a career is a personal process, requiring self-awareness and self-direction, which develops over time in meaning, tasks, and energy involved.

By applying this approach, you set individualized career goals and form a personalized action plan with strategies to reach goals and gain career fulfillment and vitality. You can use this approach to validate the wisdom of past actions that resulted in your present career path and to set new directions along different career paths.

Components of the Framework

The framework of career management for nurses is illustrated in Figure 3–1. The disks represent the three areas of information needed for career management. The divisions within the disks represent the components of the problem-solving approach. The diamond shape within each disk indicates career goals, and the lines connecting the corners of the diamonds designate key career strategies.

The three areas of information necessary to manage your career effectively are self, nursing options, and trends. These are illustrated as disks of equal size to show their equal importance. The hierarchical arrangement of the disks

Figure 3–1 Career management framework for nurses. © Frances C. Henderson and Barbara O. McGettigan.

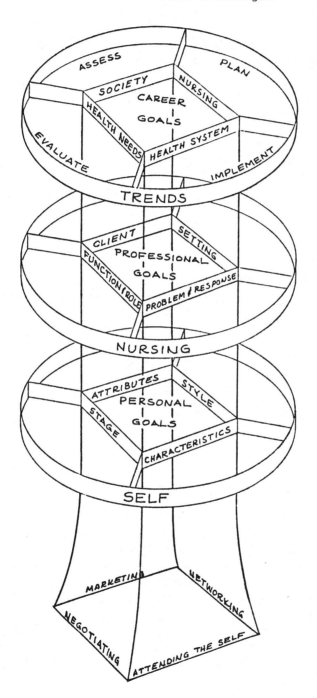

places the self at the bottom, because information about you forms the basis for career management. The fundamental consideration for selecting, changing, and developing your career is you! Your personal traits are important unique attributes, considered from several aspects, as they relate to your preference of nursing options and your consideration of the trends that will influence your career plan. The disk representing nursing options has the central focus since it interfaces with both self and trends. The topmost disk depicts the overriding effects of societal, health care, and nursing trends on nursing options and the self.

Two processes are essential to a self-directed career management approach: problem solving and use of career management strategies. The problem-solving process is illustrated in each of the three disks. The four familiar steps—assessment, planning, intervention, and evaluation—are arranged to show that assessment and planning are complementary, as are implementation and evaluation. The components of the problem-solving process hinge on career goals.

Career management strategies are depicted as major threads, which connect the four corners of the diamonds (goals). These strategies are marketing, negotiating, networking, and attending the self. They support career goals by providing approaches and techniques to apply the problem-solving process and form the support structure for other components of the framework.

The framework specifies three levels of goals to guide career prescriptions and plans of action. The three-dimensional diamond shapes depict these goals. Goals anchor career management and move from personal goals, to goals related to nursing options, to definite career goals that consider trends, the professional self, and nursing options.

Self, Nursing Options, and Trends

Gathering information about the self, nursing options, and trends can be as limited or as extensive as you choose. However, gaining adequate information related to each area promotes effective and innovative career management. Methods and sources for collecting information are discussed in Chapter 4.

The Self

Key information about the self includes personal characteristics, attributes, style, and stage. *Personal characteristics* refer to needs, values, and interests. Do you need security or recognition? Do you value achievement, financial success, or collegiality? Are your interests in the social rather than the physical sciences? Personal characteristics such as these contribute to your initial selection of a career and to your ongoing adaptation to changes in career goals.

Attributes such as your skills, special knowledge, and experience affect how well you can reach career goals. Assessing both general and nursing skills in working with people, data, or ideas, presented in Chapter 5, helps you determine how feasible various career goals are for you. You can combine special knowledge with a career option so that a personally satisfying pathway evolves. For example, Joe, a nurse with expertise and experience in interior decorating, designed critical care units to minimize client and staff stresses. Another nurse, Alma, intrigued by and knowledgeable about fashion, conducted seminars for nurse managers and executives on how to communicate their roles to their organizations through wardrobe selection. These are two of a wide variety of ways nurses combine special experience with professional knowledge and skill to formulate very unique nursing options.

Another personal aspect that refers to your approach to tasks and people is *style*. It is reflected in the way you do or say things rather than in what you actually do or say. Style can be a somewhat elusive aspect, but it is portrayed in how you learn, how you make decisions, and how you communicate. Since people as well as organizations have certain styles, assessing yours can assist you in making decisions about a setting for your practice. For instance, a nurse with a very rational and methodical approach may not be suited to a reactive, crisis-oriented health agency.

Stage influences your career goals, your expectations, and the actions that you choose to reach your goals. Stage refers to your place in the life span. It affects the meaning and importance of your career, the degree of career commitment, and the level of proficiency in your practice. The career life span extends from the point of establishing a career to the point of retiring from a career. Your position along that continuum, whether at the point of selecting a career, expanding it, reentering it, reevaluating it at mid-life, or winding down from it, strongly influences the goals you establish and the actions you take. For instance, a woman whose children have grown and left home and who has time and energies available might consider expanding her career and enroll in an educational program for a degree. On the other hand, for a single parent with two young children who is a new graduate, success in the first job is crucial and a return to school might be a poorly timed effort.

The meaning and importance of your career changes over time. In some phases of life, recreation, community involvement, or social obligations may be the focus of most of your time and energies. At other times, your career may be the central focus. Sometimes a job is something you do. At other times a career expresses who you are.

Your level of proficiency in your professional practice is an aspect of your stage in career. It influences the goals you set and the amount and kind of goal planning that you do. For example, knowing if you are at the beginner, proficient, or expert level (Benner, 1984) helps you establish realistic goals for the future. Knowing your current nursing stage also gives you a sense of self-confidence and self-acceptance and minimizes stress that can stem from inadequate understanding of the natural development of professional expertise.

Nursing Options

The second area of information needed for nursing career management is nursing options. You should know and assess these options and acknowledge their rewards and requirements.

A comprehensive assessment of your preferences for clients, practice settings, health problems, nursing functions, and roles exposes you to the richness and diversity of nursing options. Once you analyze each of these facets, you can combine them in a variety of ways. For example, Paul focused on coronary artery disease and its prevention by doing investigative work with an insurance company, analyzing the incidence and contributory factors within industrial settings, and planning appropriate intervention for target groups of clients. Jan, who had a similar focus, decided that her predominant client group was children and developed health promotion programs for school-age children for the regional heart association.

In addition to analyzing facets of nursing, you should consider the rewards and requirements involved in nursing options. Other-directed nurses considering outcomes and rewards from a personal rather than a client point of view may find this aspect difficult. But assessing whether your needs, values, and interests will be met with various options is critical to personal satisfaction, a sense of fulfillment in your career, and effective career management. Whatever you value, be it competition or collegiality, high technology or high touch, high income or personal satisfaction, the options you are now considering should closely match your personal characteristics and meet your needs or expectations.

Information about the requirements of nursing pathways is also mandatory. If you are planning to be a clinical specialist or home care administrator, investigate what education or special skills, experiences, and preparation are needed. Recognizing career prerequisites assists you in making career selections and developing career plans. In Chapter 6 you will explore nursing practice, develop several nursing options and recognize rewards and requirements for those options.

Trends

The third area of information integral to career management is trends. After you have formulated hypothetical nursing goals, you verify them or discount their viability based on an assessment of trends. A realistic career goal emerges from this assessment. For example, you may choose to practice as an ostomy nurse with adult clients in an acute care setting, but trends may project that this role has less than a 5-year viability due to shortened durations of client hospitalizations, changing approaches to medical treatment and client teaching. With this information, you can reconsider your goal and choose an option that has a likelihood of being marketable for at least 5 years. When you intentionally consider future projections in your career goal setting and planning, you are in a much better position to respond to changes as they occur. If, for example, you plan to market a specific nursing product because your trends analysis indicates that the economy will continue to remain strong over the next year or two, you will adapt your plan if those projections change. If, however, you do not consider relevant trends, you will not be able to identify important influences that impede or support goal attainment.

Key information to consider in your career management includes trends in nursing, health care, and society. Using genius predictions and projected forecasts for nursing practice, education, research, and finances guides and validates your thinking about nursing career goals. Equally important are health care trends. What are current unmet health problems and issues as well as projected increases or decreases in disease or health impairment? What direction is the health care delivery system taking? What are the future practice settings? Appreciation of broad societal trends such as industrial growth, politics, economics, and demographics enhances your perspectives in planning and managing your career. Some approaches for addressing these questions are discussed in Chapter 7.

Key Career Management Processes

Two key processes comprise the career management framework. They are a systematic problem-solving approach and career management strategies.

Systematic Problem-Solving Approach

Effective career management involves applying the problem-solving process. In the framework the components of the process—assessment, planning, implementation, and evaluation—are superimposed on each of the information areas.

Your nursing career evolves when the problem-solving process is undertaken with an appreciation of the three dimensions: you, nursing options, and trends. The process affects and is affected by this context.

Case Example: Betti

Betti Bean, RN, MS, planned to be a hospice nurse specialist, caring for clients with acquired immune deficiency syndrome (AIDS). She chose working at the National Institute of Cancer, AIDS Unit, in lieu of doctoral studies. In developing her plan she considered personal characteristics, nursing options, and future trends. Personally she realized that she learned best from direct experiences. She had economic and social obligations that allowed a 1-year rather than 3-to-5 years learning experience. Professionally she was aware of the thrust and need for doctoral preparation. She recognized, however, that the projected tenfold increase in incidence of AIDS in her geographic area over the next 3 years called for a more immediate route to specialization.

Betti's action plan, therefore, reflects her systematic application of information about herself, nursing options, and trends in problem solving for career planning. As Betti's economic and social obligations change, she will evaluate and update her plan using the same problem-solving process.

There are many benefits to assuming a problem-solving approach to career management. Problem solving provides efficiency in attaining your goals. The problem-solving process develops skills that are valuable in implementing your career. In today's competitive and fast-paced world, strategic planning is important not only for organizations and groups but for each individual faced with the challenges of survival, change, fulfillment, and self-renewal. Probably most salient, however, is the joy that results from reaching toward your self-established goals. As you make systematic decisions and choose one action over others, you relinquish the "oughts" to do what you want and what you need to do. As a result, you can relish the fulfillment of your career goals, which are personal, professionally satisfying, relevant, and enviable.

The first component of systematic problem solving involves data collection and assessment about yourself, nursing, and trends. This information guides you in formulating goals. This phase of assessment ends with development of tentative career goals. The planning step involves studying the goals and testing or evaluating their worth. Once evaluation is complete, a specific career goal is chosen. An action plan is written based on that goal.

Choosing a career goal means little without actually writing a career plan. "Unwritten plans are only dreams and it is difficult to operationalize a dream" (Stevens, 1983). Written career plans help careers happen and promote rational career decision making. A career plan, however, serves only as a guide, a road map. It can and should easily be altered as you and your circumstances change. A career plan is also a checkpoint for you to inspect and measure progress against the time frames and according to the outcomes you have established. Activities, methods, resources, and time frames are identified that will help you reach specific outcomes.

The implementation phase involves carrying out activities you have written in your plan. As you evaluate the effectiveness of your plan, ask yourself if the actions are sufficient for reaching the goal you have established or if the time frames and goal remain realistic. Are you doing what you set out to do, and are you reaching the goal? In addition, maintain awareness of the changes and trends in the nursing profession and yourself, and consider how these confirm or conflict with your current goal and plans. If your assumptions about the future prove incorrect, then you will need to rethink and perhaps realign your career goal, actions, and time frames according to your revised perceptions.

What you value and want from your career inevitably change over time. The resources you can allocate to your career and the degree of your career commitment change over your life span. Sometimes unexpected events such as divorce or illness occur. All of these changes require re-evaluation of your career direction and goals as well as your plan of action. Of course, once you attain and integrate goals, you gain increased self-awareness and then start once again to explore and reach out for additional development and search for new goals. Evaluation stems from implementation and leads to a reassessment, new goals and plans.

The problem-solving process is continual and ongoing. The steps are not distinct or separate but fluid. Assessment assists you in developing effective plans and helps you establish realistic outcomes for evaluating. Often you assess, plan, implement, and evaluate concurrently. What is essential is that you carry out all aspects of the process. Guidelines for career planning and evaluating are discussed in Chapter 8.

Career Management Strategies

Career management requires that you cultivate and apply selected strategies. Career management strategies involve putting yourself in the right place at the right time, developing the right contacts, presenting your best side, and developing your own self-portrait. Specifically, career strategies consist of four key skills: negotiating, networking, marketing, and attending the self. These are detailed in Chapter 9. These strategies assist in all aspects of career management, whether it be assessing yourself or nursing, appreciating trends, or actually implementing your career plan. Applying career management strategies also prevents and treats common career distress syndromes. The problems of career transitions and role stress are averted or alleviated with strong supports and networks, negotiating for what is needed, and giving authentic attention to the self.

Negotiating is a type of communication. You assert your needs and goals, and you make reasonable trade-offs to get where you want to be. It requires attention to verbal and nonverbal cues and a consideration of the range of possible outcomes. The optimum result of negotiation is mutual gain.

Networking refers to identifying and cultivating relationships with others for the purpose of sharing information and resources. Building a cadre of resources involves working with peers, mentors, preceptors, role models, sponsors, coaches, and counselors. Each of these resource persons serves in a different capacity vis-à-vis your career management.

Marketing means featuring your best qualities and skills—acknowledging yourself as the "product" and a potential employer as a valued "buyer." You decide the target most receptive and appropriate to you and your goals and present your strengths in a way that is most appealing to that person, group, or institution. Marketing includes effective presentation skills, resume writing, job interviewing, and the gaining of recognition.

Attending the self is another fundamental career management strategy. It means developing self-awareness, assuming self-direction of your career, and administering self-care. Constant and conscious self-awareness as well as attention to internal direction are essential for effective career management.

Career management strategies are akin to handling a beautiful piece of artwork. Creating artwork, like creating a career plan, requires one set of skills and knowledge. But once that art piece or career plan is created, a different set of skills is needed. The art product must be carefully wrapped, shipped and received, and displayed appropriately. Similarly, a career plan must be carefully prepared and displayed for you to realize your maximum potential.

Like the problem-solving approach to career management, the use of career management strategies is undertaken within the key areas of self, nursing options, and trends. This means you select and acquire the strategies that are appropriate and meaningful to you, the profession, and the future as you see it. In addition, career strategies are selected and used in ways that are appropriate to your realistic nursing career goals. For instance, your background may be presented in a resume for certain positions but require a curriculum vita for others. A preceptorship may be appropriate in learning agency-specific expectations, while a sponsor may be essential to advancing within a corporation. Networks must be strong, negotiating skills flexible, marketing adept, and attending the self authentic in managing your career effectively to attain your career goals.

Goals

In the framework of career management for nurses, three levels of goals are depicted and related to each of the areas on which you collect information: self, nursing options, and trends. Personal goals represent your individual aspirations, values, and considerations of life stage and lifestyle. Personal goals become evident from your self-assessment; they reflect what is important to you regardless of a specific field or professional considerations.

Professional goals convey your preferences among nursing options and emerge from your analysis of key dimensions of self and nursing. Professional goals are still somewhat hypothetical, or tentative, in that they express the functions, roles, and other practice aspects you believe will address and integrate your personal profile and professional preferences. You then investigate the anticipated influence of projections for the future on the tentative professional goals you have developed. After final analysis, career goals emerge from a consideration of how trends interface with professional and personal goals. At this point, your career goals represent several highly probable directions that seem practical and preferable to you.

Career planning ensues once several possible career goals become evident from your exploration and assessment of yourself, nursing, and trends. Career planning starts with actually deciding on one career goal and ends with establishing an action plan to reach that goal. You decide on your career goal by reality testing and by weighing outcomes of various goals. Reality testing is similar to what Tiedeman and Miller-Tiedeman (1984) call a "crystallization" process. By reading, touring, and conducting informational interviews you ascertain the chances that tentative goals or options have of really addressing your personal needs and goals. You identify the actual consequences or rewards of the tentative options that are appealing to you.

After reality testing various career goals, you are ready to weigh probable outcomes and choose one direction, a specific goal. The choice process involves listing the outcomes of various options, the probability of these outcomes occurring, and rating the importance or value of these outcomes to you. A career goal is chosen that has the greatest value in relation to the probabilities of the outcomes actually occurring (Herr & Cramer, 1979). The goal you finally establish is a realistic nursing career goal written as a specific statement of direction and purpose. Your realistic nursing career goal details what you want to do, why, where, with whom, and by what point in time. The nursing career goal directs your plan and guides its implementation; it allows you to make your nursing career operational. Specific guidelines for choosing your career goal and designing your career plan are presented in Chapter 8.

Relationships and Interrelationships of Ideas Within the Career Management Framework

The career management framework displays the multidimensional relationship among three data areas, two key processes, and three levels of goals. The processes of problem solving and use of career strategies are embedded within the data areas of the self, nursing options, and trends. Thus, these processes should be carried out with an awareness and understanding of all three areas. Implementing these processes simultaneously influences the amount and type of data and the career goals that result.

The framework highlights the complex and dynamic nature of career management. Career management is not a simple linear action taken at one point in time. It is not merely matching yourself with an occupation. It is a complex process, involving information gathering, decision making, planning, and implementing an array of strategies. The process is dynamic, with constant interplay and adjustment between you, nursing options, and trends and your use of a systematic problem-solving approach and career management strategies.

A balance among all components of the framework is desirable for optimal results. Balance is maintained when all elements dynamically interface: self mirrors nursing options, and nursing options reflect trends. Effective problem solving allows a true integrity and consistency between the self, nursing, and trends. Strategies also maintain a balance and integrity between career and personal and professional goals.

If there is a shift in awareness or emphasis on any one element to the detriment of others, the balance is impaired. An uneven implementation of career management strategies or inadequate problem solving will tip the balance and hamper career management. Readjustment and realignment are ongoing aspects of career management. The more skilled you are with the process, the quicker you can make necessary adjustments. In addition, the more you interrelate the processess with self, nursing options, and trends, the more sophisticated and fine-tuned your career management becomes. A career managed with a high degree of problem solving and career management strategies results in the realization of desired career goals.

The starting point for any plan is gathering information. In order to make this career management framework work for you, you will have to determine the most appropriate methods and resources for gathering information about yourself, nursing options, and trends.

References

Benner P: *From Novice to Expert,* pp. 13–38. Menlo Park, CA: Addison-Wesley, 1984.

Herr E, Cramer S: *Career Guidance Through the Life Span,* pp. 77–82. Boston: Little, Brown, 1979.

Stevens K: *Power and Influence: A Source Book for Nurses,* pp. 189–190. New York: Wiley, 1983.

Tiedeman D, Miller-Tiedeman A: Career decision making: An individualistic perspective. In: *Career Choice and Development,* p. 208. Brown D, Brooks L (editors). San Francisco: Jossey-Bass, 1984.

4 Gathering Information

FRANCES C. HENDERSON
BARBARA O. McGETTIGAN

Information is a key component of the career management framework; its collection and analysis form the first of four steps in the problem-solving process. Information, both as content and as a process step, is illustrated in the nursing career management framework (see Figure 3–1). According to the framework, three areas of data, or information, are necessary to manage your career: self, nursing options, and trends. Gathering information in these three areas helps you make informed new career decisions or validate previous ones.

Criteria

Information is most useful if it is accurate, current, and adequate. Accuracy refers to validity. How extensive is the supporting evidence for the information? Is the information based on research, personal experience, or on just one incident? Consider the credentials, education, and scope of experience of the person making statements or providing the information—the more unbiased the origin, the better the resource. Bias may be present if the source has a vested interest. For example, an agency recruiter may skew images and information about the agency to attract staff or students.

Rapid changes in the body of nursing knowledge and nursing practice compel you to monitor the currency of information. The lag time between the formulation of information and its dissemination in the literature is a case in point. What you read in current publications often reflects knowledge formulated within the last 5 years. Fortunately, computer technology is gradually reducing this time lag; however, a 5-year range is still the suggested guideline for currency of information.

Information is adequate if it is sufficient in quantity and scope for you to formulate an opinion. For example, data about the clinical nurse specialist role obtained by interviewing two specialists in just one agency is limited in quantity and scope. It is restricted to responsibilities defined by one agency. Whenever possible, interview persons who work in different agencies or locations to broaden your information base and give you an opportunity to compare responses.

In order to gather adequate information, let your purpose guide the extent of your inquiry. For example, when you are weighing one or two specific options, you need details about such areas as satisfaction and stress, lines of accountability, specific functions, salary, and work schedule. But when you are exploring various options, general questions on setting, role, and practice suffice. The extent of information gathered should also be established by what is practical for you. How much time can you allocate? How available and accessible are resources in the library, health facility, or community? Do you have contacts? The critical consideration is how much information you need to be comfortable and confident with the nursing career dimensions and options you develop and the career goal you establish.

Methods

Methods for gathering information vary depending on purposes and your learning or interpersonal styles. If you are primarily a social person who learns best by direct hands-on experience, you might select experiential methods such as part-time work, shadowing a nurse, or conducting volunteer projects. On the other hand, if you are analytic or an observer, reading current literature, observing through job-site visits, or attending classes might work best for you. After completing a series of self-assessment exercises, including learning style and interpersonal style (discussed in Chapter 5), you will better be able to select methods that suit you.

Different methods suit different purposes. Some methods such as writing and introspection work well for assessing yourself. Observation and active experimentation are effective when collecting information about nursing options. Trends are best determined by talking with others and reading. Six methods for gathering information are presented here. They are reading, talking, observing, writing, introspection, and active experimentation. You are strongly encouraged to use a variety of methods most natural to your learning and interpersonal styles and appropriate to your purposes.

Reading

Reading is a most useful method of gathering information especially if you are a self-directed learner or if you favor reading as a learning mode. You may browse through nursing magazines and related periodicals, or you may choose a more systematic approach, using manual index searches or computer searches. Nursing indexes include the *International Nursing Index* and the *Cumulative Index to Nursing and Allied Literature.* Other indexes, such as *Index Medicus, Hospital Literature Index* or abstracts in nutrition, psychology, child development, and other nursing-related fields may be useful. Two major on-line data bases include the National Library of Medicine (NLM) MEDLINE and the Educational Resources Information Center, commonly called ERIC. Articles, conference proceedings, studies, and reports accessible through these methods contain a wealth of information about nursing and trends.

Other printed resources that will enhance your investigative efforts are reference books, self-help guides, assessment inventories, brochures, or pamphlets. Self-help guides and some assessment inventories may be useful in accumulating information about yourself. Read to find out what nurses and non-nurses are writing about that is applicable to nursing, the health care field, and areas that interest you. Also read to learn about current nursing issues and future trends in nursing and health care. Reading often will inspire an innovative or creative approach for you to match your personal characteristics with specific nursing options.

Data from reading ranges from general to specific. For example, it can help you determine what kinds of positions appear most often and in what area of the country, or it can point out major nursing and health care issues.

Talking

If your preferred style is social, you can glean information about yourself, your present and future career plans, nursing options, and trends by talking with peers, mentors, sponsors, or preceptors. For example, what do others like about you and what do they indicate that you do well? You can weigh this input against your perceptions of yourself. Seeing yourself as others see you often is a most-revealing exercise. Although the range of results may vary, this practice can provide you with helpful information on how your behavior reflects your beliefs. The strategy of seeing yourself through another's eyes can also provide positive reinforcement for behaviors that are important to you.

Networking   Networking is an exciting approach to gathering information through talking. Networking among groups of individuals with common or related interests is consistent with an enterprising style. Networking is informal communication with others for the purpose of exchanging essential or desired information about subjects of mutual interest. It can be viewed as a series of communication links, each link representing a different but related information source as illustrated in Figure 4–1.

In addition to enhancing your own visibility, networking can help you determine the major leaders in a field of interest and their career paths. You

Figure 4–1 Communication links of networking.

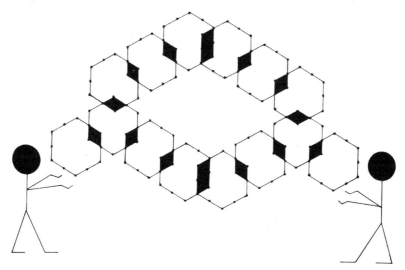

can find out how positions of interest to you are obtained and to what organizations or groups persons in these positions belong.

The following list of actions will help you use networking as an information-gathering approach:

1. Avail yourself of opportunities to participate with others informally at conferences, conventions, workshops, on committees, and in similar activities.

2. Make a note (mental or written) of names and information you want to pursue. For example, request a business card and write a descriptive note on it that will remind you of the person or topic.

3. Have your own business card available to exchange with others as appropriate. If you do not have a card, offer your name, address, and phone number to the person with whom you wish to establish contact.

4. As you mingle with others, note position titles and organization affiliations associated with names.

5. Listen to introductions of speakers, but also check your written program for additional biographic information.

6. Initiate conversation by introducing yourself first.

7. Let others know what your interests, experiences, and aspirations are and maintain an awareness of their responses.

8. Listen carefully to the interests, values, and experiences of others.

9. Take the opportunity to talk further with those who share your interests, values, and goals or those who have had or who are seeking experiences similar to your own.

10. Develop a sensitivity for the kinds of information that interest you now as well as for that which might serve some future need. (You may find use for some information several months after you have collected it.)

11. Be prepared to respond to others who may approach you for information. After all, networking is a reciprocal process, involving the exchange of information.

12. Employ patience and persistence in developing and using your networking skills. You seldom can expect to master a skill on the first try. Therefore, analyze your strategies, consider what worked well for you, and identify what skills you would like to improve and how you might do so.

Networking expedites the exchange of information and encourages the refinement of loosely held ideas. It is a key strategy for gathering information as well as for managing your career. (Networking as a career management strategy is discussed in Chapter 9.)

Informational Interviewing Informational interviewing is an approach to gathering data that works especially well if your preferred style is investigative. It is a structured method of posing questions and exploring career options. It is a key strategy for obtaining input about a variety of positions and related information. A job interview, on the other hand, focuses on one specific position in a selected organization and is based on intent to secure that position. Informational interviewing as a strategy for exploring career options can contribute greatly to preparation for later job interviews.

Most of the skills used in client assessment interviews can also be used to gather information about nursing career options and trends. The application of open-ended and direct questions as well as observation of nonverbal communication remains the same.

It will be helpful to your interviewee if you share some essential information about yourself and the type of information you need. For example, ''I am exploring nursing options and am interested in hearing what you do in your position as . . .,'' or ''I am interested in your view of nursing and health care trends related to positions as . . . .''

Open-ended questions require an explanatory response. For example, asking ''What do you like most about your roles and responsibilities as a . . . ?'' rather than, ''Do you like what you do?'' requires more than a yes or no response. Direct questions provide you with specific information and make effective use of interview time. For example, asking ''How did you achieve the qualifications for the position of . . . ?'' limits answers to the most relevant information or opens the communication to general exploration.

Since nonverbal communication is an important expression of feelings, you need to observe your interviewee's expressions of enthusiasm, pride, satisfaction, or reticence. Observe for incongruence between verbal and nonverbal communication. The nurse who relates excitement and enthusiasm for a position in a dull tone hardly sounds convincing.

Timing is essential to the ultimate effectiveness of any communication, including informational interviews. Be sure to arrange in advance a mutually convenient time and a suitable duration for the interview. If a specific duration of time is hard to predict, ask your interviewee how much time she or he has for sharing information with you. Consider the times most feasible for interviewing the person(s) you have selected and the amount of time you feel you will need to gather necessary information.

A setting that is mutually agreed on, conveniently located, and free of unnecessary interruptions is conducive to talking and listening. Using a conference room, lounge, quiet dining room, or an office where phone calls and interruptions can be handled by someone else may be suitable. Some find a park, living room, study, or a quiet space in a restaurant appropriate and more personal.

Select nurses who are practicing in or involved with the roles that are congruent with your goal. If you are considering self-employment in a creative venture independent of a formal organization or are creating an innovative position for yourself within an organization, you need information from persons whose needs and interests will be served by your new position. You also need knowledge about the roles and responsibilities of the position you are seeking.

In addition to choosing who you should interview, you must determine how many persons to interview. Whenever possible, interview at least three people because this will broaden your information base. It will also give you an opportunity to compare responses. The uniqueness of the options you are pursuing may limit the number of persons available. If you are considering more innovative pursuits, a process of successive data-gathering sessions from a number of persons will help you form and refine your own ideas.

In your interview ask questions that are broad enough to give you complete data, but specific enough to provide information related to your areas of interest. Questions related to options and trends in nursing may focus on (a) roles, responsibilities, and qualifications of various areas of practice or positions that interest you; (b) the range of possible intrinsic and extrinsic rewards; and (c) trends that may affect the supply and demand of nurses with these specific qualifications and interests.

In addition to informational interviewing, consider holding informal data-gathering sessions with nurses and other health care professionals. Often valuable information is gleaned over lunch or at social activities where communication is spontaneous and unstructured.

The process of talking with others, then, is an extremely useful and often appropriate information-collecting method. Variations of approach include talking with others personally, networking, or informational interviewing, depending on your preferred style. The range of data available through this method is endless. The data gathered helps solve career problems and establish long-term relationships that can serve you well in all phases of managing your career.

Writing

The writing method of gathering information is best suited to obtaining information about yourself. Approaches are personal, such as keeping a diary, and objective, such as maintaining a career journal.

Expressing your thoughts, feelings, pleasant and unpleasant experiences, plans, and dreams in a journal or diary is one strategy for getting in touch with yourself. It enhances the process of identifying recurring life themes and important self-characteristics. If the availability of significant others with whom to share thoughts and plans is limited or if you like to refine your ideas before sharing them, writing and reexamining them periodically is helpful. Even if you do not like to write, it is easy to write about a subject on which you are an expert.

There are numerous formats of diaries and journals, but a simple blank book or any note pad will get you started quickly and easily. You may write more than once a day, daily, or at infrequent intervals. Date your entry, and begin by writing whatever thoughts come to mind, letting them flow through your fingertips and onto the page. You may find yourself writing lists, amusing anecdotes, a lengthy narrative with no punctuation, or poetry.

You may prefer to keep a career journal rather than an entirely personal one. The purpose of a career journal is to provide a means for gathering data about your career that can assist you in designing, refining, or validating your career plan. One suggestion for such a journal is to specify a period of time such as 1 to 4 weeks, during which you record and analyze aspects of your current position. Aspects could include tasks, roles, responsibilities, and expectations. Position title and the functions a person actually performs often differ; thus a record that compares position description and performance evaluations with actual experiences helps you grasp the "real" job specifications and clarify your feelings and interpretations about your current position.

If you are feeling dissatisfied with your current position, keeping a career journal can provide significant data to analyze the reasons for your dissatisfaction. You may find other uses for information from your journal such as setting priorities, time management, and short- or long-term career planning.

The process of gathering information about yourself through writing is an enlightening experience. You will find many uses for such data when weighing personal characteristics against preferred nursing options, when selecting career management strategies, and when considering the effect of current or future trends on your career goals and plan.

Introspection

Introspection is a valuable method for gathering information about yourself. It is a natural inclination for the person who learns best through activities that involve feeling. Looking deep inside yourself for your innermost thoughts and feelings can reveal valuable data related to your personal characteristics. It often helps you identify a specific pattern of success or achievement or, equally valuable, obstacles that constrain your attainment of specific personal goals.

Introspection is best achieved in an environment such as a quiet park, a beach, or your own personal space in which you do your best thinking, where you can turn your energies inward and explore your innermost thoughts. Along your inward journey, ask yourself questions: Who am I really? Am I pleased with who I am? Am I pleased with where I am at this point in my life? Where do I want to be in my life and in my sense of myself 6 months from now? In 1 year, 2 years, 5 years, or more? What do I like about me? What do I do best? What are my five most important beliefs? What are the five things I most like to do? As you begin to know your innermost self, think of other questions to ask; let the questions and answers flow spontaneously. The more you learn about yourself, the better you will be able to match your identified personal attributes to your preferred nursing options and nursing career goals.

Observing

Observing others may be formal or informal. Daily nursing practice involves systematic and automatic observation of clients' behaviors. By applying this same method to collecting data related to your career goals, you can observe persons in positions to which you aspire in a number of ways. For example, in university settings observing experienced professionals is an essential component of role development. With the increasing emphasis on preceptor experiences, internships, externships, and mentor systems, individuals are encouraged to use observational methods and arrange their own observation experiences. Arranging site visits to observe different settings such as tertiary care settings, surgery centers, or industrial health offices will also provide much information about some differences and similarities in nursing options.

You may choose to make informal observations of persons in positions of interest to you, accumulating information about activities in which they are involved. Your observations will add to your data base what you like most about these activities, what you like least, and how these persons demonstrate enthusiasm. Your observations will also attune you to any obvious signs of stress that may be associated with these roles and responsibilities. Arranging to shadow a nursing faculty member or a discharge coordinator at work to gain insight into specific nursing roles are examples of this approach.

You can also obtain information when attending meetings of fellow professionals. For example, observe how others make contacts, enhance their visibility, and involve themselves in networking with others. You can learn ways to enhance your own visibility and assertiveness by simply observing others.

Active Experimentation

Active experimentation is an information-gathering method of actually assuming various roles and responsibilities. It is well suited to those who have a learning style preference for direct trial and analysis. Approaches may be short-term such as negotiating with a manager to exchange roles for a few days. This gives you an opportunity to appreciate the responsibilities and feel of the manager's role in your setting in a limited but realistic fashion. Long-term approaches include volunteering or agreeing to serve in an acting position in your agency. Securing a part-time position in a setting compatible with your career goals is another approach to the use of active experimentation. All of these approaches would clarify specific nursing roles and settings, enabling you to accumulate information about your responses, preferences, and the skills needed or already gained.

Information Sources

Information sources are plentiful, becoming even more so in our information-focused society. The challenge is to select those that will provide you with adequate, accurate, and current information. A major source of information is you. Significant others also help you shape your perceptions. People, or human, resources are a cornerstone of information. Other sources are print media, professional nursing and nursing-related organizations, and visual media such as videotapes.

People Resources

People resources take a variety of forms, depending on the roles they assume in relation to you. Examples include mentors, counselors, sponsors, coaches, and role models.

Mentors.   Mentors use a variety of approaches to help individuals discover and maximize potential. Mentors may be colleagues, relatives, friends, teachers, counselors, or supervisors. They may or may not be nurses. Mentors are best identified by how they help you and by how they make you feel about yourself. Mentors help you by listening actively to your dreams and aspirations and reflecting what you communicate both verbally and nonverbally for your reexamination. They help you by asking pertinent questions that allow you to elaborate on your answers. They make you feel cared about, challenged, and supported. Although some may equate mentorship with coaching, sponsorship, or specific guidance and support within an organization, mentorship here refers to a highly personal, significant enabling relationship that is not limited to hierarchical structure nor to a specific organization.

The mentor/protégé relationship, described by Kelly (1984), is based on a patron-mentorship system. This type of relationship is characterized by the power and influence of the mentor and the willingness of the mentor and protégé to devote intensive time and effort over relatively long periods to shared professional goals. Other variations of mentor relationships may not involve a hierarchical relationship within the same organizational structure and may vary both in time and intensity. What nurse mentors and those they guide seem to share are common interests, commitment to their profession, and a willingness to risk being open, honest, and innovative. Special characteristics of effective nurse mentors are caring and nurturing qualities and their political astuteness. Effective nurse mentors visualize nursing's future and thus the need for well-prepared leaders whose career paths they can help shape.

Career-oriented nurses are increasingly interested in what a mentorship is and how it can be part of their professional lives. Nurses who are successfully planning their careers often identify one or more mentors who are significant to them in this process.

Advantages of mentorship are its self-perpetuating relationship supportive of personal and professional development, and its flexibility in accomodating individual changes as well as changes in circumstances. Disadvantages of mentorship include the tendency to feel overwhelmed by challenges or to become overextended in meeting unrealistic expectations.

Counselors.   Counselors help you explore personal traits, needs, interests, and skills by interviewing and administering standardized tests. They interpret test results, suggest a variety of options, and may help you develop a career plan. Numerous career and vocational counseling services can be found in your community. Most of these services are provided for the general public, but a few career counseling services designed exclusively for nurses are beginning to appear. Career counseling also is provided through centers located on college and university campuses or affiliated with local community associations such as Young Men's/Women's Christian Associations.

Sponsors, Coaches, and Role Models.   Sponsors, coaches, and role models are key people sources of information and influence within organizations. The power of sponsors is their influence on promoting those whom they oversee within a specific work environment or institution. Sponsors have the organizational power to open doors for the potential nurse executive (Scott, 1984). They are also a primary resource for information such as the language, actions, and behaviors of the corporate culture. Coaches are usually supervisors who provide an appraisal of your performance and information related to your career progression within the organization. They provide strong encouragement to help you secure promotional opportunities. Role models typically provide you with information through observing them as an image of where, what, and how you would like to be. You imitate these desired behaviors using active experimentation.

People are a rich and rewarding information resource. They provide you with essential information by sharing direct experiences, past experiences, and personal and professional insights. They can also share their predictions about future trends.

Print Media

Libraries are a primary source of print media. These include public, specialty, hospital, college and university campus libraries as well as your personal library of journals, reference books, publications.

Professional groups or organizations also are important sources of print media about nursing and trends. For instance, the National Student Nurses' Association, The American Journal of Nursing Company, and Intermed Communications, Inc. publish annual career planning guides. Many career opportunity profiles are included in these guides. The National League for Nursing publishes an array of brochures and directories with information about nursing, nursing educational programs, and available scholarships. The American Nurses' Association also has a wealth of information on certification for nurses, standards for various types of nursing practices, and statistical data about nurses.

Other sources of print media include international and national health organizations (Table 4–1 in Chapter Appendix) and nursing organizations. Voluntary health agencies, such as the American Red Cross, The American Heart Association, the American Cancer Society, the American Diabetes Association or any of the other disease-oriented organizations, which can be contacted at chapters in the community, have much information about health problems and issues as well as nursing opportunities within their agencies. Other organizations such as the World Health Organization (WHO), Peace Corps, and People to People Health Foundation (Project HOPE) provide information for those interested in opportunities in underserved areas or developing countries.

Examples of international and national nursing organizations include the International Council of Nursing, National League for Nursing, and the American Nurses' Association. Others are listed in Table 4–2 in the Chapter Appendix. Regional nursing organizations include the Western Interstate Commission on Higher Education (WICHE), Southern Council on Collegiate Education For Nursing (SCCEN), New England Organization of Nursing (NEON), Mid-Atlantic Regional Nursing Association (MARNA), and the Midwest Alliance In Nursing (MAIN). Regional organizations (Table 4–3 in Chapter Appendix) publish and disseminate information on the status of nursing and trends by geographic region and workshop proceedings and reports of long-term projects on issues related to nursing.

State Boards of Registered Nursing (Table 4–4 in Chapter Appendix) provide information about particular states, nursing practice regulations and statutes, and educational institutions accredited by them. For information about hospitals, the American Hospital Association publishes a directory that describes the capacity, ownership, specialties, and address of hospitals in the United States.

Professional Organizations

Professional nursing organizations sponsor conferences, conventions, and workshops, where several information-gathering opportunities are available. While the presentations are a source of data, you can also use these events as an opportunity to network. State nurses' associations are listed in Table 4–5 in the Chapter Appendix. More than 60 organizations representing nursing specialists, types of nursing practice, and special services for nurses are listed in Table 4–6 in the Chapter Appendix. These organizations often can assist you by identifying practitioners in your locale to interview about qualifications and particulars of their specialties. National health organizations, state nurses' associations, and local nursing associations provide similar information regarding general practice.

The wide array of information sources provided here includes various types of people resources, selected sources of print media, and over 200 organizations and regulatory agencies that offer a variety of information and services related to nursing. Given this array, you need only select those that will most meet your needs. Knowing how to gather and organize your information is the next useful step.

Helpful Hints for Gathering Information

Some helpful hints will assist you in planning and organizing your information-gathering approaches. Allow yourself adequate lead time to choose the people or sources you need to contact. Write letters or obtain necessary directions to gain access to information. Follow letters with phone calls to reiterate your intent and enthusiasm. It is helpful to have a set of 5 × 8 cards (like those used when doing a literature search) on which to keep your data categorized and organized. Use your cards to make notes related to areas of inquiry. A sample data-collection file card is illustrated in Figure 4–2.

Figure 4–2 Sample data collection file card.

Career goal: _____

Data collection method: Read _____ Talk _____ Write _____

                                 Introspect _____ Observe _____

Data source: People _____ Print _____

                 Organization _____

Specific name, title _____

Date _____

     Content of questions   Data or findings

        (key words)

1.

2.

3.

4.

5.

6.

To insure the accuracy of your information sources, make a note of the positions, background, and experiences of the authors of print media, presenters at conferences, and other people resources. Note the dates of articles or conversations. Establish the timeliness of print media by noting publication dates. The currency of information from people resources can be determined by the extent to which your people resources are attuned to current issues, trends, and key local or national leaders.

You alone decide whether the information you collect is adequate, since the extent of your information-gathering efforts will be guided by your purpose. You need information about yourself to formulate personal goals, about nursing options to direct your focus in establishing possible career goals, and about nursing trends as the critical context within which to make realistic decisions and plans.

The methods and sources, or "how to's," of collecting information are key components of career management. Chapters 5, 6, and 7 guide you in the "what" of data gathering. Specific questions will become clearer as will the types of information needed to answer questions and formulate personal and career goals.

References

Directory of Nursing Organizations. *AJN*, (April) 1985; 4:493–500.

Kelly L: From the president. *Sigma Theta Tau Reflections,* (April/May) 1984, p. 1.

The AJN Guide: A Review of Nursing Career Opportunities in 1983, pp. 40–41. New York: American Journal of Nursing, 1982.

Scott P: Executive career planning. *Nurs Econ,* (Jan/Feb) 1984; 2:58–63.

Specialty nursing organizations. *Career Information Services.* New York: National League for Nursing, (in press). 1–2.

Appendix

Table 4–1 International and National Health Organizations

American Association of Diabetes Educators
Box 56, N Woodbury Rd
Pitman, NJ 08071

American Association for Respiratory
   Therapy
1720 Regal Row
Dallas, TX 75235

American Cancer Society
777 Third Ave
New York, NY 10017

American Diabetes Association
600 Fifth Ave
New York, NY 10020

American Heart Association
840 North Lakeshore Dr
Chicago, IL 60611

American Hospital Association
840 North Lakeshore Dr
Chicago, IL 60611

American Lung Association
1740 Broadway
New York, NY 10019

American Medical Society
535 North Dearborn St.
Chicago, IL 60610

American Public Health Association
1015 15th St NW
Washington, DC 20005

American Red Cross
17th and D Streets NW
Washington, DC 20006

American School Health Association
PO Box 708
1521 South Water St
Kent, OH 44240

American Society of Childbirth
PO Box 16159
7113 Lynnwood Dr
Tampa, FL 33687

American Urological Association Allied
6845 Lake Shore Dr
PO Box 9397
Raytown, MO 64133

Association of the Care of Children In
   Hospitals
3615 Wisconsin Ave NW
Washington, DC 20016

Joint Commission on Accreditation of
   Hospitals
875 North Michigan Ave
Chicago, IL 60611

National Institutes of Health
900 Rockville Pike
Bethesda, MD 20205

National Kidney Association
2 Park Ave
New York, NY 10016

Office of Human Development Service
Office of Policy and Legislation
200 Independence Ave SW
Washington, DC 20201

Pan American Health Organization
525 23rd St NW
Washington, DC 20037

Peace Corps
806 Connecticut Ave NW
Rm P-301
Washington, DC 20526

People to People Health Foundation (Project
   HOPE)
Millwood, VA 22646

US Office of Personnel Management
1900 E St NW
Washington, DC 20415

US Public Health Service
Dept of Health and Human Services
5600 Fishers Lane
Rockville, MD 20857

World Health Organization
Avenue Appia, 1211
Geneva 27, Switzerland

From Directory of Nursing Organizations, *AJN* (April) 1985; 4:493, with permission.

Table 4–2 International and National Nursing Organizations

Alpha Tau Delta National Fraternity for Professional Nurses 14631 N Second Dr Phoenix, AZ 85023	International Council of Nurses 3 place Jean Marteau 1201 Geneva, Switzerland
American Association of Colleges of Nursing 1 Dupont Circle Suite 530 Washington, DC 20036	National League for Nursing 10 Columbus Circle New York, NY 10019-1350
American Nurses' Association 2420 Pershing Rd Kansas City, MO 64108	National Student Nurses' Association 10 Columbus Circle New York, NY 10019-1350
American Organization of Nurse Executives 840 North Lakeshore Dr Chicago, IL 60611	Sigma Theta Tau National Honor Society of Nursing 1100 Waterway Blvd Indianapolis, IN 46202
International Committee of Catholic Nurses and Social Assistants Palazzo S Calisto 1-00120 Cittadel Vaticano, Itly	World Federation of Neurosurgical Nurses 286 W 2nd St Morrestown, NJ 08057

From Directory of Nursing Organizations, *AJN* (April) 1985; 4:493, with permission.

Table 4–3 Regional Nursing Organizations

Mid Atlantic Regional Nursing Association Teachers College Columbia University Box 146 525 W 120 St New York, NY 10027	Southern Council of Collegiate Education for Nursing 1340 Spring St NW Atlanta, GA 30309
Midwest Alliance in Nursing Room 108-BR Indiana University 1226 W Michigan St Indianapolis, IN 46223	Western Interstate Commission for Higher Education PO Drawer P Boulder, CO 80302
New England Organization of Nursing c/o EDC 55 Chapel St Newton, MA 02160	

From Directory of Nursing Organization, *AJN* (April) 1985; 4:496, with permission.

Table 4–4   State Nurses' Associations

Alabama State Nurses' Association 360 North Hull St Montgomery, AL 36197	Indiana State Nurses' Association 2915 North High School Rd Indianapolis, IN 46224
Alaska Nurses' Association 237 E Third St Anchorage, AK 99501	Iowa Nurses' Association 215 Shops Bldg Des Moines, IA 50309
Arizona Nurses' Association 4525 N 12th St Phoenix, AZ 85014	Kansas State Nurses' Association 820 Quincy St Room 520 Topeka, KS 66612
Arkansas State Nurses' Association 117 S Cedar Little Rock, AR 72205	Kentucky Nurses' Association 1400 S First St PO Box 8342, Station E Louisville, KY 40208
California Nurses' Association 1855 Folsom St Room 670 San Francisco, CA 94103	Louisiana State Nurses' Association 712 Transcontinental Dr Metairie, LA 70001
Colorado Nurses' Association 5453 E Evans Pl Denver, CO 80222	Maine State Nurses' Association 283 Water St PO Box 2240 Augusta, ME 04330
Connecticut Nurses' Association 1 Prestige Dr Meriden, CT 06450	Maryland Nurses' Association 5820 Southwestern Blvd Baltimore, MD 21227
Delaware Nurses' Association 2466 Capitol Trail Newark, DE 19711	Massachusetts Nurses' Association 376 Boylston St Boston, MA 02116
District of Columbia Nurses' Association 5100 Wisconsin Ave NW Suite 306 Washington, DC 20016	Michigan Nurses' Association 120 Spartan Ave East Lansing, MI 48823
Florida Nurses' Association Box 6985 Orlando, FL 32853	Minnesota Nurses' Association 1821 University Ave Room N-377 St Paul, MN 55104
Georgia Nurses' Association 1362 W Peachtree St NW Atlanta, GA 30309	Mississippi Nurses' Association 135 Bounds St Suite 100 Jackson, MS 39206
Hawaii Nurses' Association 677 Ala Moano #601 Honolulu, HI 96813	Missouri Nurses' Association 206 East Dunklin St PO Box 325 Jefferson City, MO 65102
Idaho Nurses' Association 1134 N Orchard #8 Boise, ID 83706	Montana Nurses' Association 715 Getchell Box 5718 Helena, MT 59604
Illinois Nurses' Association 20 N Wacker Suite 2520 Chicago, IL 60606	

Table 4–4   *Continued*

Nebraska Nurses' Association 941 O ST Suite 711 Lincoln, NE 68508	Rhode Island State Nurses' Association H.C. Hall Building (South) 345 Blackstone Blvd Providence, RI 02906
Nevada Nurses' Association 3660 Baker Lane Reno, NV 89509	South Carolina Nurses' Association 1821 Gadsden St Columbia, SC 29201
New Hampshire Nurses' Association 48 West St Concord, NH 03301	South Dakota Nurses' Association 1505 S Minnesota Suite 6 Sioux Falls, SD 57105
New Jersey State Nurses' Association 320 W State St Trenton, NJ 08618	Tennessee Nurses' Association 1720 West End Bldg Suite 400 Nashville, TN 37203
New Mexico Nurses' Association 525 San Pedro NE Suite 100 Albuquerque, NM 87108	Texas Nurses' Association 300 Highland Mall Blvd Suite 300 Austin, TX 78752
New York State Nurses' Association 2113 Western Ave Guilderland, NY 12084	Utah Nurses' Association 1058 E Ninth S Salt Lake City, UT 84105
North Carolina Nurses' Association Box 12025 Raleigh, NC 27605	Vermont State Nurses' Association 500 Dorset St Middleschool S Burlington, VT 05401
North Dakota State Nurses' Association Greentree Square 212 N Fourth St Bismarck, ND 58501	Virginia Nurses' Association 1311 High Point Ave Richmond, VA 23230
Ohio Nurses' Association 4000 E Main St PO Box 13169 Columbus, OH 43213	Washington State Nurses' Association 83 S King St Suite 500 Seattle, WA 98104
Oklahoma Nurses' Association 6414 N Santa Fe Suite A Oklahoma City, OK 73116	West Virginia Nurses' Association 512 D St Charleston, WV 25303
Oregon Nurses' Association 9700 SW Capitol Hwy Suite 200 Portland, OR 97219	Wisconsin Nurses' Association 6117 Monona Dr Madison, WI 53716
Pennsylvania Nurses' Association 2578 Interstate Dr PO Box 8525 Harrisburg, PA 17105	Wyoming Nurses' Association 1603 Capitol Ave Majestic Building Room 305 Cheyenne, WY 82001

From Directory of Nursing Organizations, *AJN* (April) 1985; 4:496–500, with permission.

Table 4–5   State Boards of Registered Nursing

Alabama Board of Nursing
500 Eastern Blvd
Suite 203
Montgomery, AL 36117

Alaska Board of Nursing
Dept. of Commerce and Economic
  Development
Pouch D
Juneau, AK 99811

Arizona Board of Nursing
5050 N 19th Ave
Phoenix, AZ 85015

Arkansas Board of Nursing
4120 W Markham
Suite 308
Little Rock, AK 77205

California Board of Nursing
1030 13th St
Sacramento, CA 95814

Colorado Board of Nursing
State Services Bldg, Room 132
1525 Sherman St
Denver, CO 80203

Connecticut Board of Nursing
150 Washington St
Hartford, CT 06106

Delaware Board of Nursing
Margaret O'Neil Building
Federal and Court Streets
Dover, DE 19901

District of Columbia Board of Nursing
614 H Street NW
Washington, DC 20001

Florida Board of Nursing
111 E Coastline Dr
Suite 504
Jacksonville, FL 32202

Georgia Board of Nursing
166 Pryor St SW
Suite 400
Atlanta, GA 30303

Hawaii Board of Nursing
Box 3469
Honolulu, HI 96801

Idaho Board of Nursing
Hall of Mirrors
700 W State St
Bosie, ID 83720

Illinois Department of Registration and
  Education
320 W Washington St
Springfield, IL 62786

Indiana Board of Nurses' Registration
  and Nursing Education
964 N Pennsylvania
Indianapolis, IN 46204

Iowa Board of Nursing
1223 East Ct
Des Moines, IA 50319

Kansas Board of Nursing
PO Box 1098
503 Kansas Ave
Suite 330
Topeka, KS 66601

Kentucky Board of Nursing
4010 Dupont Circle
Suite 430
Louisville, KY 40207

Louisiana Board of Nursing
907 Pere Marquette
150 Baronne St
New Orleans, LA 70112

Maine Board of Nursing
295 Water St
Augusta, ME 04330

Maryland Board of Examiners of Nurses
201 W Preston St
Baltimore, MD 21201

Table 4–5 *Continued*

Massachusetts Board of Registration in Nursing 100 Cambridge St Room 1521 Boston, MA 02202	New Mexico Board of Nursing 5301 Central NE Suite 905 Albuquerque, NM 87108
Michigan Board of Nursing PO Box 30018 Lansing, MI 48909	New York Board of Nursing State Education Dept Cultural Education Center Albany, NY 12230
Minnesota Board of Nursing 717 Deleware St SE Minneapolis, MN 55414	North Carolina Board of Nursing Box 2129 Raleigh, NC 27602
Mississippi Board of Nursing 135 Bounds St Suite 101 Jackson, MS 39206	North Dakota Board of Nursing 418 E Rosser Bismarck, ND 58501
Missouri Board of Nursing 3523 N Ten Mile Dr Box 656 Jefferson City, MO 65102-0656	Ohio Board of Nursing Education and Nurse Registration 65 S Front St Room 509 Columbus, OH 43215
Montana Board of Nursing Dept of Commerce 1424 Ninth Ave Helena, MT 59620	Oklahoma Board of Nurse Registration and Nursing Education 2915 N Classen Blvd Suite 524 Oklahoma City, OK 73106
Nebraska Board of Nursing Box 95007 Lincoln, NE 68509	Oregon Board of Nursing 1400 SW Fifth Ave Room 904 Portland, OR 97201
Nevada Board of Nursing 1135 Terminal Way Suite 209 Reno, NV 89502	Pennsylvania Board of Nursing Box 2649 Harrisburg, PA 17105
New Hampshire Board of Nursing State Office Park South 101 Pleasant St Concord, NH 03301	Rhode Island Board of Nursing Cannon Health Building 75 Davis St Providence, RI 02908
New Jersey Board of Nursing 1100 Raymond Blvd Room 319 Newark, New Jersey 07102	

Table 4–5   *Continued*

South Carolina Board of Nursing 1777 St Julian Pl Suite 102 Columbia, SC 29204	Virginia Board of Nursing 517 W Grace St PO Box 27708 Richmond, VA 23261
South Dakota Board of Nursing 304 S Phillips Ave Suite 205 Sioux Falls, SD 57102	Washington Board of Nursing Box 9649 Olympia, WA 98504
Tennessee Board of Nursing Bureau of Manpower & Facilities 283 Plus Park Blvd Nashville, TN 37219–5401	West Virginia Board of Examiners for Registered Nurses 922 Quarrier St Embleton Bldg, Room 309 Charleston, WV 25301
Texas Board of Nursing 1300 E Anderson Land Bldg C, Suite 225 Austin, TX 78752	Wisconsin Board of Nursing PO Box 8936 Room 174 Madison, WI 53708
Utah Division of Registration-Board of Nursing Heber M Wells Building 160 E 300 S PO Box 45802 Salt Lake City, UT 84145	Wyoming Board of Nursing 2223 Warren Ave Suite One Cheyenne, WY 82002
Vermont Board of Nursing Redstone Building 26 Terrace St Montpelier, VT 05602	

From Directory of Nursing Organization, *AJN* (April) 1985; 4:496–500.

Table 4–6 Specialty Nursing Organizations

Aerospace Medical Association Flight Nurse
Section ASMA
PSC Box 3009
APO NY 09223

American Academy of Ambulatory Nursing
Administration
N Woodbury Rd
Box 56
Pittman, NJ 08071

American Assembly for Men in Nursing
c/o College of Nursing
Rush University
600 S Paulina—474-H
Chicago, IL 60612

American Association for Critical Care
Nurses
One Civic Plaza
Newport Beach, CA 92660

American Association of Industrial Nurses
PO Box 478
Dallas, TX 75221

American Association of Nephrology Nurses
N Woodbury Rd
Box 56
Pittman, NJ 08071

American Association of NeuroScience
Nurses
22 S Washington St
Suite 203
Park Ridge, IL 60068

American Association of Neurosurgical
Nurses
625 N Michigan Ave
Suite 1519
Chicago, IL 60611

American Association of Nurse Anesthetists
216 Higgins Rd
Park Ridge, IL 60068

American Association of Nurse Attorneys
PO Box 5564
Washington, DC 20016

American Association of Occupational
Health Nurses
3500 Piedmont Rd NE
Atlanta, GA 30305

American College of Nurse-Midwives
1522 K St NW
Suite 1120
Washington, DC 20005

American Holistic Nurses' Association
PO Box 116
Telluride, CO 81435

American Indian/Alaska Native Nurses'
Association, Inc
PO Box 1588
Norman, OK 73070

American Society of Ophthalmic Registered
Nurses, Inc
PO Box 3030
San Francisco, CA 94119

American Society of Plastic and
Reconstructive Surgical Nurses
N Woodbury Rd
Box 56
Pittman, NJ 08071

American Society of Post-Anesthesia Nurses
2315 Westwood Ave
Suite 1
PO Box 11083
Richmond, VA 23230

Association for Practitioners in Infection
Control
505 E Hawley St
Mundelein, IL 60060

Association of Nurses Practicing
Independently
21 Spruce St
Dept NL
Dansville, NY 14437

Table 4–6   *Continued*

Association of Operating Room Nurses 10170 E Mississippi Ave Denver, CO 80231	National Association for Practical Nurse Education and Service 10801 Pear Tree Lane Suite 151 St Louis, MO 63134
Association of Pediatric Oncology Nurses Pacific Medical Center PO Box 7999 San Francisco, CA 94120	National Association of Hispanic Nurses 2014 Johnston St Los Angeles, CA 90031
Association of Rehabilitation Nurses 2506 Gross Point Rd Evanston, IL 60201	National Association of Nurse Recruiters 30 Woodland Dr Churchville, PA 18966
Commission on Graduates of Foreign Nursing Schools 3624 Market St Philadelphia, PA 19104	National Association of Orthopaedic Nurses N Woodbury Rd Box 56 Pittman, NJ 08071
Dermatology Nurses' Association N Woodbury Rd Box 56 Pittman, NJ 08071	National Association of Pediatric Nurse Associates and Practitioners 1000 Maplewood Dr Suite 104 Maple Shade, NJ 08052
Emergency Nurses' Association 666 North Lake Shore Dr Suite 1131 Chicago, IL 60611	National Association of Physician's Nurses 9401 Lee Hwy Suite 210 Fairfax, VA 22031
Lesbian α Gay Nurses' Alliance 801 E. Harrison Suite 105 Seattle, WA 98102	National Association of Quality Assurance Professionals, Inc Dept NL 1800 Pickwick Ave Glenview, IL 60025
Gerontological Nursing 844 West End Annapolis, MD 21401	National Association of School Nurses, Inc PO Box 1300 Lamplighter Lane Scarborough, ME 04074
International Association for Enterostomal Therapy, Inc One Newport Pl Suite 970 Newport Beach, CA 92660	National Black Nurses' Association, Inc PO Box 18358 Boston, MA 02118
National Association for Health Care Recruitment PO Box 93851 Cleveland, OH 44101	

Table 4–6 *Continued*

National Federation of Licensed Practical Nurses, Inc 214 South Dr PO Box 11038 Durham, NC 27703	Nurses' Christian Fellowship 233 Langdon St Madison, WI 53703
National Flight Nurses' Association Life Flight Allegheny General Hospital 320 E North Ave Pittsburgh, PA 15212	Nurses' Coalition for Action in Politics 1030 15th St NW Suite 408 Washington, DC 20005
	Nurse Consultants' Association PO Box 25875 Colorado Springs, CO 80936
National Intravenous Therapy Association, Inc 87 Blanchard Rd Cambridge, MA 02138	Nurses' Educational Funds, Inc 555 W 57th St New York, NY 10019
National Nurses' Society on Addictions 2506 Gross Point Rd Evanston, IL 60201	Nurses' House, Inc 10 Columbus Circle New York, NY 10019
National Nurses' Society on Alcoholism PO Box 7728 Indian Creek Branch Shawnee Mission, KS 66207	Nurses in Transition PO Box 14472 San Francisco, CA 94114
Nurses' Alliance for the Prevention of Nuclear War Box 319 Chestnut Hill, MA 02167	Nurses Now PO Box 5156 Pittsburgh, PA 15206
	Oncology Nursing Society 3111 Banksville Rd Pittsburgh, PA 15216
Nurses' Association of the American College of Obstetrics and Gynecologists 600 Maryland Ave SW Suite 200 East Washington, DC 20024	Otolaryngology and Head/Neck Nurses c/o Warren Otologic Group 3893 E Market St Warren, OH 44484

Table 4–6   *Continued*

Public Health Nursing/American Public Health Association 1015 Fifteenth St NW Washington, DC 20005	The Society for Nursing History Nursing Education Dept Box 150 Teachers College Columbia University New York, NY 10027
Society for Advancement in Nursing, Inc Cooper Station, Box 307 11th St and 4th Ave New York, NY 10003	
Society for Parenteral and External Nutrition 1025 Vermont Ave NW Suite 8110-Dept N 81 Washington, DC 20005	Transcultural Nursing Society College of Nursing University of Utah 25 S Medical Dr Salt Lake City, UT 84112
Society for Peripheral Vascular Nursing 1070 Sibley Tower Rochester, NY 14604	United Nurses' Associations of California 170 W San Jose Ave Suite 102 Claremont, CA 91711
Society for Research in Nursing Education School of Nursing, N319Y University of California, San Francisco Third and Parnassus Ave San Francisco, CA 94143	United Nursing Home Association 16400 Southcenter Pkwy Suite 410 Seattle, WA 98188

From Specialty Nursing Organizations. *Career Information Services.* New York: National League for Nursing (in press); *The AJN Guide 1983*, AJN Company, NY, 1982; Directory of Nursing Organizations, *AJN* (April) 1985; 4:494–495, with permission.

5 Assessing Yourself

FRANCES C. HENDERSON

Assessing yourself is an active process of specifying your personal characteristics, attributes, style, and stage related to managing your career in nursing. Your needs, values, and interests are among your personal characteristics; attributes include your knowledge, experience, and skills; style refers to your approach to tasks and people; and stage indicates your place in your life and career spans. Because personal growth and development tend to parallel career development, this chapter focuses on self-assessment, the first step of a developmental approach to making the best possible use of your potential as a nurse. In subsequent chapters, you will apply the results of your self-assessment to determine practice options, roles, and career management strategies best suited to your profile.

You Are Your Own Greatest Resource

Self-Assessment

Just as client assessment guides the planning and implementation of nursing care, self-assessment guides career planning and the implementation of these plans. Likewise, as reassessment of clients is essential in determining the effects of nursing actions, periodic self-reassessment helps determine the effects of the activities of implementing career plans.

You are your own greatest resource! If you are to grow and develop as a unique individual and as a nurse, collecting information that will help you determine or confirm who you are is the place to start.

Who Are You?

You are a unique individual, an arrangement of interrelated component human parts that form a whole person. You are a composite of biologic, psychologic, social, cultural, and spiritual ingredients. This blend of ingredients allows you to play the roles of your life: spouse, parent, son or daughter, citizen, student, teacher, nurse. But which of these roles best defines you? If asked who you are, do you say, "I'm a nurse," or "I'm a teacher"? What is your usual response? Ask yourself now and consider your answer.

Ideal Self Versus Real Self

An image of the self as perfect in any one of several life roles is one definition of the ideal self. Examples include the perfect parent, loving spouse, self-sufficient adult, par golfer, 300 bowler, or model nurse. Images of self are based on strongly held ideals. These ideals are shaped by a combination of social forces, institutional influences such as family, church, and school, role models, and a myriad of life experiences. If early life experiences were clouded by temporary deprivation of basic needs, aspirations of wealth may be an ideal. The childhood influences of a close, supportive family often engender the same ideal for one's own family. Nurses' ideals may well be shaped by influential instructors, supervisors, peers, or the rigorous process of nursing education. Parental ideals often emulate the parent who is considered perfect. Throughout your life, input from those close to you and from society shape and reshape how you see yourself.

Your real self is what you are now, an individual whose self-image is shaped by the various roles you assume. What is your ideal image of yourself? How does it compare with your real self? By looking at yourself as an individual, taking into consideration your ideal self and your real self, you can identify your strengths and aspirations, which you later will relate to your career goals and career management. Congruence between real self and ideal self can be a significant source of inspiration when effectively managing your nursing career.

Self and Society

Political, technical, economic and demographic forces as well as social institutions such as family, church, and school determine ideals, personal values, and practices, thus influencing self-perceptions. These self-perceptions are altered continuously by the natural phenomena of social change. Realistic self-perception in view of social change requires individual flexibility and stability. Problems arise when self-perception remains static, owing to previously held but no longer relevant values, often resulting in a limited self-concept. When attempts to adjust to rapid social change result in overextension of self, adapting in several directions simultaneously, a grandiose self-concept and overtaxing

Figure 5–1 Balance of personal reality and self-concept.

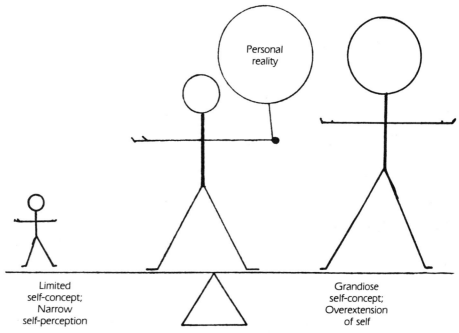

Limited
self-concept;
Narrow
self-perception

Grandiose
self-concept;
Overextension
of self

of personal resources may be the consequence. Either narrow or overextended self-perception can cause you to lose sight of your personal reality. The challenge is to seek a balance between the two extremes (Figure 5–1).

Your perception of who you are is influenced by others significant to you and by society at large. Assessing the extent to which you really know yourself can help you confirm the priorities associated with your identity and reconfirm your perception of yourself. Self-awareness, discussed in Chapter 2, is a key requisite to self-assessment. The more aware you are of yourself and your personal dimensions (see Exercise 2–3), the more receptive you are likely to be to an in-depth assessment of your personal characteristics, attributes, style, and stage.

Personal Characteristics

Personal characteristics reflect your values, interests, and needs. This section consists of a series of self-assessment activities that will help you identify some of these characteristics, which you may apply in subsequent chapters on career planning and career management.

Value

Your values are prized modes of conduct that define your behavior and desires. Cherished values you are likely to affirm publicly are highly regarded beliefs that you act on repeatedly. How do values affect your career? If you value independence are you a nurse practitioner or a consultant, or are these among your career aspirations? If you value a sense of accomplishment, is it evident in your career position? These strong beliefs form your personal goals, career goals, and sense of self-esteem.

Your life values are most likely reflected in the kinds of contributions you make through your performance as a nurse and the kinds of rewards you want to receive for your efforts. It is helpful to consider this as you develop or refine your career goals and plans.

Exercise 5–1   Your Most Cherished Values

Listed here are 20 life values identified by Hagberg and Leider (1982). First read through the list, thinking of your values as modes of conduct that define your behavior and desires. Then reread it and rank the values in the spaces provided from 1 (most cherished) to 20 (least cherished).

a.   Achievement (sense of accomplishment/promotion)   _____

b.   Adventure (exploration, risks, excitement)   _____

c.   Personal freedom (independence, making your own choices)   _____

d.   Authenticity (being frank and genuinely yourself)   _____

e.   Expertness (being good at something important to you)   _____

f.   Emotional strength (ability to handle inner feelings)   _____

g.   Service (contribute to satisfaction of others)   _____

h.   Leadership (having influence and authority)   _____

i.   Money (plenty of money for things you want)   _____

j.   Spirituality (meaning to life, religious beliefs)   _____

k.   Physical health (attractiveness and vitality)   _____

l.   Meaningful work (relevant and purposeful job)   _____

m.   Affection (warmth, caring, giving and receiving love)   _____

n.   Pleasure (enjoyment, satisfaction, fun)   _____

o.   Wisdom (mature understanding, insight)   _____

p.   Family (happy and contented living situation)   _____

q.   Recognition (being well-known, praised for contribution)   _____

r.   Security (having a secure and stable future)   _____

s.   Self-growth (continuing exploration and development)   _____

t.   Intellect (having a keen, active mind)   _____

In the spaces provided write the five values you most cherish in order of their priority.

1.   _____

2.   _____

3.   _____

4.   _____

5.   _____

Interests

Your interests are the things you enjoy. Interests in this context have been grouped by Holland (1973) and modified by others, including Johansson (1980), Bolles (1981), and Hagberg and Leider (1982), into three broad categories of things, data, and people with six general themes (Table 5–1).

Table 5–1 Interest Categories and General Themes

Category	General Theme
Things	Realistic
Data	Investigative; artistic; conventional
People	Enterprising; social

The six general themes describe characteristics of people in the population at large based on work by Holland (1973). If you have a wide range of interests, you will no doubt identify with activities in each of the theme areas. The wider your range of interests, the more flexible you are likely to be. In a time of rapid technical and social change this flexibility, if judiciously used, can be an asset. On the other hand, identifying a narrow range of interests consistent with one specific theme may enhance understanding yourself in relation to activities congruent with this theme; in some cases it may help you focus on what you want to do.

Exercise 5–2   A Modified Interests Inventory

Sets A to F in this exercise are descriptors from similar inventories by Hagberg and Leider, Johansson, and Bolles. Twelve activities, which describe things you may enjoy, are listed in each set. As you read each list, use a check mark to indicate the activities that reflect your interests. Use a number in the appropriate column to indicate the extent of your interest from 1 (low) to 3 (high). Add your interest scores and place the total in the score box at the end of each list. An interpretation of your scores follows the sets of exercises.

Set A	Most describes you (√)	Interest		
		Low 1	Moderate 2	High 3
1. Biking				
2. Cooking				
3. Dancing				
4. Designing objects				
5. Adjusting equipment				
6. Operating equipment				
7. Woodworking				
8. Needleworking				
9. Sailing				
10. Swimming				
11. Running				
12. Skiing				
Score total				

Set B	Most describes you (√)	Interest		
		Low 1	Moderate 2	High 3
1. Assessing others				
2. Using logic				
3. Experimenting				
4. Observing				
5. Clarifying problems				
6. Researching				
7. Surveying				
8. Analyzing				
9. Diagnosing problems				
10. Testing ideas				
11. Critiquing				
12. Evaluating				
Score total				

Set C	Most describes you (√)	Interest		
		Low 1	Moderate 2	High 3
1. Applying theory				
2. Creating new ideas				
3. Developing models				
4. Designing visuals				
5. Creating works of art				
6. Directing productions				
7. Drawing				
8. Composing music				
9. Acting				
10. Predicting				
11. Taking pictures				
12. Writing poetry				
Score total				

84

Set D	Most describes you (√)	Interest		
		Low 1	Moderate 2	High 3
1. Caring for others				
2. Coaching				
3. Counseling				
4. Editing				
5. Listening				
6. Designing educational materials				
7. Leading groups				
8. Negotiating				
9. Writing letters				
10. Writing reports				
11. Reading				
12. Translating				
Score total				

Set E	Most describes you (√)	Interest		
		Low 1	Moderate 2	High 3
1. Initiating ideas				
2. Planning changes				
3. Taking risks				
4. Assigning tasks				
5. Setting standards				
6. Coordinating activities				
7. Implementing policies				
8. Managing conflict				
9. Speaking in public				
10. Competing in games				
11. Telling stories				
12. Using humor				
Score total				

Set F	Most describes you (√)	Interest		
		Low 1	Moderate 2	High 3
1. Keeping deadlines				
2. Carrying things out in detail				
3. Making contracts				
4. Organizing records				
5. Classifying data				
6. Filing				
7. Processing forms				
8. Inventorying				
9. Keeping financial records				
10. Managing budgets				
11. Allocating resources				
12. Following through on others' instructions				
Score total				

Interpretation

The maximum interest themes score is 36. Following is the scoring grid that explains which of the sets of activities illustrate specific themes. Write your scores in the appropriate spaces.

Interest Themes Scoring Grid

Set	Theme	Score
A	Realistic	
B	Investigative	
C	Artistic	
D	Social	
E	Enterprising	
F	Conventional	

Use the following key to interpret the extent of your interests (high, moderate, or low) according to the sum of your scores.

Interest Themes Scoring Key

Score range	Interpretation
30–36	High
26–29	Moderate
22–25	Low

Are you surprised by the results of this exercise? Are the activities in which you have a high interest consistent with your perception of yourself? Are your interests mostly grouped in one or two theme areas or are they distributed over several themes? Reflect on how your high-interest themes are manifested in your personal and career goals and in your choice of nursing as a career.

Needs

Needs are required by nature or circumstance for survival, safety, security, belonging, personal growth, and self-actualization. Like values, they are determined by early life experiences. For example, physiologic needs for survival vary according to climate and availability of the essentials: food, clothing, and shelter. Safety and security needs are shaped by the extent to which they are or are not met from earliest infancy. According to Maslow's hierarchy of needs, basic survival and security needs must be met before social needs, ego needs, and self-actualization are realized. In Chapter 2 you completed an exercise to help you identify the level of needs met by your work in nursing and to determine the extent to which you are satisfied with that level. In Exercise 5–3 you will identify and rank your needs from a comprehensive list.

Exercise 5–3   Identifying Your Needs

Read the following list of 25 needs and check those that are most essential to you. Then rank those selected, beginning with 1 as most essential. If you have particular needs other than those listed, space is provided at the end of the list for you to write them. Include any additions in your priority rating.

Needs	Priority rating	Needs	Priority rating
1. Independence	_____	3. Being well-known	_____
2. Self-respect	_____	4. Creativity	_____

	Needs	*Priority rating*		*Needs*	*Priority rating*
5.	Beauty	_____	18.	Sense of accomplishment	_____
6.	Money	_____	19.	Meaningful work	_____
7.	Orderliness	_____	20.	Being good at something	_____
8.	Belonging	_____	21.	Ability to handle inner feelings	_____
9.	Pleasure	_____	22.	Genuineness	_____
10.	Insight	_____	23.	Continual self-development	_____
11.	Intelligence	_____	24.	Secure and stable future	_____
12.	Giving and receiving love	_____	25.	Spirituality	_____
13.	Intimacy	_____		_____	_____
14.	Physical vitality	_____		_____	_____
15.	Altruism	_____		_____	_____
16.	Being praised	_____		_____	_____
17.	Excitement	_____			

As you rated your needs, did some of them sound similar to your priority list of cherished values (Exercise 5–1)? Several items on both lists are the same. When your cherished values, needs, and interests are consistent with and match your role and responsibilities in nursing, you have a greater likelihood of attaining career satisfaction. Conversely, identifying mismatches can assist you in your career planning and management. Table 5–2 lists matched values and needs; Case Example A is a sample summative profile of

Table 5–2 Match Between Values and Needs

Values	Needs	Values	Needs
Achievement	Sense of accomplishment	Physical health	Physical vitality
Adventure	Excitement	Meaningful work	Meaningful work
Personal freedom	Independence	Affection	Giving and receiving love
Authenticity	Genuineness	Pleasure	Pleasure
Expertness	Being good at something	Wisdom	Insight
Emotional strength	Ability to handle inner feelings	Family	Intimacy
Service	Altruism	Recognition	Being well-known
Leadership	Being well-known	Security	Secure and stable future
Money	Money	Self-growth	Continual self-development
Spirituality	Spirituality	Intellect	Intelligence

personal characteristics. Exercise 5–4 gives you an opportunity to construct your own profile.

Case Example A: Sample Profile of Personal Characteristics

Values	Needs	Interest themes
Family	Independence	Investigative (36)
Self-growth	Self-respect	Social (36)
Intellect	Meaningful work	
Emotional strength	Continual self-development	
Spirituality		

I greatly value my family and our home. Self-growth, a keen active mind, emotional strength, and my own inner spirituality are cherished values, which are in some ways matched with my needs. Independence ranks first as my highest need. I have been a single parent head of household for 15 years, therefore this is no surprise. Independence is matched with the high value I place on members of my family and my responsibility for them. I need to respect myself, engage in meaningful work, which nursing is for me, and I need to pursue my own self-development perpetually. What makes me unique is my level of comfort with this combination of values and needs in relation to my interests. I scored equally high on both the investigative and social themes. I love working with people and data; I am a "psych" nurse, and I especially love teaching, reading, and writing.

Exercise 5–4   Profile of Your Unique Personal Characteristics

According to the results of your assessment of your personal characteristics (Exercise 5–1), how would you describe yourself? In the columns that follow write your five most cherished values, the five essential needs you gave highest priority, and the interest themes in which you scored 22 and above.

Values	Needs	Interest themes
_____	_____	_____
_____	_____	_____
_____	_____	_____
_____	_____	_____
_____	_____	_____

In the space provided write a comprehensive statement describing your personal characteristics.

_____

_____

_____

_____

_____

What significant patterns did you identify that make you unique? You will have an opportunity to use this information later in this chapter as well as in subsequent chapters.

Attributes

As a nurse you possess a rich reservoir of knowledge, experience, and skill from a variety of resources and situations. Your candid and in-depth assessment of the scope of your knowledge, experience, and skill is an essential part of your personal profile. It helps form your multi-dimension image. Nursing attributes become so integrated in nurses' daily living that they are seldom isolated or measured. Even when completing an application for a position or writing a resume, we often omit significant attributes.

Knowledge and Experience

Benner (1984) differentiates among practical knowledge (know-how), theoretic knowledge, and knowledge that is an integral part of expertise. Theoretic knowledge establishes causal relationships between events, enabling theorists to examine systematically a series of events as a basis for prediction. Theoretic knowledge and practical experience combine to form expertise, which is the intuitive ability, or skill, to view situations in their entirety. Expertise is not an easily measured attribute. When interviewing for positions, you may therefore be asked to describe examples of situations that demonstrate your expertise or respond to a hypothetical situation posed by the interviewer. For example, if you are a candidate for a teaching position, you might be asked to present a sample instructional module.

Self-assessment of the gestalt of your knowledge, experience, and skill is difficult to present as a paper and pencil exercise. One method is to compile a list, or comprehensive portfolio, of your educational background, work experiences, and achievements. Table 5–3 presents a suggested table of contents for such a comprehensive portfolio.

Table 5–3 Comprehensive Portfolio: Table of Contents

I. Educational background
II. Licenses and credentials
III. Career review
IV. Organizational memberships
V. Publications and presentations
VI. Professional achievements and accomplishments
VII. Appendixes

Your portfolio may be contained in a folder with pockets, a ring binder, a folder with brads to hold your papers and index tabs for easy access, or a series of color-coded and labeled folders or file cards. Select the type of organizer that works best for you. Most importantly, keep it close at hand and use it as a place to file additional documents. You will find it a handy reference on many occasions.

Exercise 5–5 Compiling a Comprehensive Portfolio

In the space provided, complete the following information as instructed.

Education Beginning with high school, list all institutions attended, their locations, attendance dates, degrees or certificates earned, and study majors.

Institution	Location	Dates attended (mo/yr)		Degree	Study major
		From	To		

Special Knowledge   If your learning was achieved by special means (for example, continuing education, on-the-job training, independent study), indicate how, what, and where you obtained it.

_____

_____

_____

_____

Licenses, Credentials, and Certificates   List your licenses, credentials, and certificates (for example, LVN or RN License, teaching credential, and Nurse Practitioner or Nurse Midwife certificates). Include the state license number, credential or certificate number, and any expiration dates.

_____

_____

_____

_____

Organization Memberships   List names of organizations to which you belong. Include offices held and committees of which you are (or have been) a member.

_____

_____

_____

_____

Publications   List articles, papers, books, and other print media such as policies and procedures or patient teaching modules you have developed. (List publications by title, date, and publisher.)

_____

_____

_____

_____

_____

_____

Special Achievements List your significant professional achievements such as honors or awards received, special recognition, or unique projects in which you have participated.

_____

_____

_____

Nursing Career Review Chronicle your nursing career, beginning with your first position as a nurse and ending with your present one. Complete the items requested in a cluster. Use as many clusters as necessary to record your nursing career (three are provided here, but they are easily duplicated).

1. Position title (first nursing position):

    _____

    Beginning month and year: _____

    Total number of years in this position: _____

    Roles and functions (use descriptive, action-oriented phrases; for example, "Staff Nurse III: Planned and coordinated care for clients on a 30-bed adult surgical unit")

    _____

    _____

    _____

    Influence on career (rate the positive, $+1$ to $+5$, or negative, -1 to -5, influence of this position on your career by circling the appropriate number):

    $+5$ $+4$ $+3$ $+2$ $+1$ 0 -1 -2 -3 -4 -5

    How acquired (indicate whether by application and selection process, promotion, referral, self-created, or other means):

    _____

    Ending month and year: _____

    Name and address of employer: _____

    _____

    Name of immediate superior: _____

2. Position title:

    _____

    Beginning month and year: _____

Total number of years in this position: _____

Roles and functions:

_____

_____

_____

How acquired: _____

Influence on career:

+5   +4   +3   +2   +1   0   −1   −2   −3   −4   −5

Ending month and year: _____

Name and address of employer: _____

_____

Name of immediate superior: _____

3.   Position title:

_____

Beginning month and year: _____

Total number of years in this position: _____

Roles and functions:

_____

_____

_____

How acquired: _____

Influence on career:

+5   +4   +3   +2   +1   0   −1   −2   −3   −4   −5

Ending month and year: _____

Name and address of employer: _____

_____

Name of immediate superior: _____

Appendixes   Your portfolio appendixes are crucial. Table 5–4 includes a list of suggested appendixes to include in your portfolio. Even if you have thrown away your old college catalogs, try to obtain copies of descriptions of courses you have taken. If your career plan includes pursuing additional education, you will find these a valuable resource to document prior learning. Your portfolio should contain copies of *all* your transcripts.

Table 5–4   Portfolio Appendixes

A. Transcripts (all educational institutions)

B. Course descriptions of postsecondary and graduate courses

C. Certificates of completion of education

D. Awards

E. Current continuing education certificates

F. Information on renewal of organization memberships

G. Published materials (where appropriate, such as articles and papers)

H. Completed applications for positions

I. Completed applications for admission to educational institutions

J. Performance evaluations

K. Letters of commendation

L. Letters of recommendation

M. Curriculum vitae or resume

N. Other related documents

Although an official copy is required for educational institutions and for some positions, it is wise to have your own copy available for reference. Keeping completed applications for positions or for admission to educational institutions will save you time and energy when filling out similar applications or replacing an original should it inadvertently be lost. A file of awards, published materials, performance evaluations, letters of recommendation, and letters of commendation will allow you to acknowledge your achievements and successes periodically, especially when you need to reinforce your self-confidence, take stock of your accomplishments, or include them in your innovative marketing package. Copies of your resumes and curriculum vitae make periodic updates easier and less time-consuming.

Your portfolio can become a central repository for reminders of dates for license or membership renewals and for certificates of completion for continuing education courses. The contents are a valuable resource for resume and curriculum vitae development. Once you have compiled a portfolio, update it annually or whenever important personal or professional information changes. As you collect additional documents specifically related to your career progression, index or label them appropriately and place them in your portfolio.

Skills

Nursing skills are assessed in a number of ways—from the concrete, such as what you can do at a psychomotor level, to the abstract, such as what you do intuitively based on a combination of applied knowledge and prior experiences. They are also assessed according to the same theme categories as interests presented earlier in this chapter: people, data, and things. Exercises 5–6 and 5–7 assess your skills according to level of proficiency and preference.

Using the Dreyfus Model of Skill Acquisition, Benner (1984) researched the performance of RNs, new graduates, and experienced nurses. As they advance in performance, nurses change both in actual skill and in their awareness of the context of practice situations. Reliance on principles gives way to use of concrete perceptions and past experiences. Nurses move from differentiation and analysis to synthesis and evaluation, so that whole situations are experienced rather than multiple tasks. A gestalt is perceived, forming the basis for establishing priorities.

The axiom that states "a nurse is a nurse is a nurse" no longer applies because of the levels of proficiency found within nursing practice: novice, advanced beginner, competent, proficient, and expert (Benner, 1984). Characteristics of proficiency levels from novice to expert (Table 5–5) are based on Benner's work.

Table 5–5   Characteristics of Proficiency Levels

Level	Characteristics
Novice: Stage 1	No experience related to situations in which they are expected to perform; rely on rules to guide actions (for example, nursing students, new graduates, and nurses entering a clinical setting in which they have had no experience with that client population, role, or specific setting)
Advanced beginner: Stage 2	Evidenced by performance based on limited recurring experiences and concrete guidelines from experienced others; perform basic assessment skills but are limited in abilities to discern the relative importance of the results (for example, nursing students nearing completion of nursing education, new graduates, or reentry nurses in preceptorship, internship, or externship programs)
Competent: Stage 3	Experience on the job in stable situations for at least 2 years; systematically solve problems and deliberately analyze situations (for example nurses in their third year of work experience in clinical settings with similar clients and situations)
Proficient: Stage 4	Evidenced by the ability to perceive situations with speed and flexibility; perceive situations as wholes due to ability to apply reflections based on previous experiences (for example, nurses who have worked with similar client populations for 3 to 5 years)
Expert: Stage 5	Having immediate and intuitive grasp of situations and perceptions based on experience and mastery of previous complex situations (for example, nurses who have 5 or more years of work experience with similar client populations and settings)

Adapted with permission from Benner, P: *From Novice to Expert.* Menlo Park, CA: Addison–Wesley, 1984

Exercise 5–6 Your Level of Proficiency

Think of your level of proficiency in nursing skills as a continuum from novice (1) to expert (5). Circle the number or place between the numbers on the following scale to indicate your perceived proficiency level.

1	2	3	4	5
Novice	Advanced beginner	Competent	Proficient	Expert

In the following space describe a recent experience in which you demonstrated your level of proficiency.

_____

_____

_____

_____

_____

_____

This exercise is intended to be subjective and introspective. In the hustle and bustle of nurses' everyday lives, there is little time and few guidelines for a self-assessment of the extent of your comprehensive skills expertise. Unlike procedural skills, proficiency level is the gestalt of your knowledge, experience, and skills as a nurse. It gives you a sense of direction and anticipation, in terms of planning what you want to do at what level, and a projected time line for your growth and development related to specific expertise.

Skill preferences are often evident in the type of positions nurses choose. Psychiatric nurses probably have a higher preference for activities with people and a social theme, whereas nurses involved in clinical research presumably have a higher preference for activities associated with the investigative theme. In Exercise 5–7 you will identify your skill preferences and the extent to which you include them among your attributes and in your career.

Exercise 5–7 Your Skill Preferences

Twenty-one statements are listed here that identify certain nursing skills. For each statement, indicate the extent to which you prefer performing that skill by circling the appropriate number in the column on the right (3 indicates high preference, 1 is low preference).

Skill Items	*Preference*		
1. Counseling clients and families individually or in groups	1	2	3
2. Caring for groups of clients	1	2	3
3. Applying humor therapy to relieve the tensions of people with pain	1	2	3
4. Supervising nurses and clients to realize institutional or unit goals	1	2	3
5. Selling or urging purchase of nursing products or services	1	2	3
6. Having a consultation service that advises on and provides staff for care of postsurgical coronary clients	1	2	3
7. Mentoring or coaching nursing staff on their role in implementing the nursing process	1	2	3
8. Instructing clients on self-care measures	1	2	3
9. Interpreting monitors for rapid detection of client problems	1	2	3
10. Using dance therapy with a client group	1	2	3
11. Working with equipment and supplies used in client care	1	2	3
12. Designing computer-assisted nursing education programs	1	2	3
13. Coordinating staffing for nursing service	1	2	3
14. Developing budgets for nursing units	1	2	3
15. Compiling epidemiologic data	1	2	3
16. Developing nursing models or theories	1	2	3
17. Designing new ways to deliver nursing services	1	2	3
18. Producing a nursing television spot for a public relations office	1	2	3
19. Researching clients' responses to pain and to alternative nursing treatment modalities	1	2	3
20. Auditing charts against established criteria for standards of care	1	2	3
21. Serving on staff of a statewide nursing project for education/service analysis of nurses' competencies	1	2	3

Scoring

Use the following steps to calculate the score of your nursing skill inventory.

Step 1: Enter the number you circled for each statement in the appropriate space for each of the three categories.

Step 2: Add your preference scores for each category of statements, then divide your total score by the number of statements in that category.

A. People skills (instructing, caring, selling, managing)

Statement: 1   2   3   4   5   6   7   8

Your preference score: _____

Your total score = _____ ÷ 8 = _____

B. Mechanical or technical skills (working with things and motion)

Statement: 9   10   11   12

Your preference score: _____

Your total score = _____ ÷ 4 = _____

C. Data skills (working with numbers, creating something new, or abstracting information)

Statement: 13   14   15   16   17   18   19   20   21

Your preference score: _____

Your total score = _____ ÷ 9 = _____

Does your inventory indicate one dominant category of skills? A score of 3 designates high preference, 2 moderate preference, and 1 low preference. Fill in your scores for each category of this inventory from Exercise 5–7 and for your interest themes from Exercise 5–2.

Summary of Scores

Nursing skills inventory		Interest themes score		
Category	Your score	Theme	Set	Your score
People skills	_____	Enterprising	E	_____
		Social	D	_____
Mechanical or technical skills	_____	Realistic	A	_____
Data skills	_____	Investigative	B	_____
		Artistic	C	_____
		Conventional	F	_____

Interpretation.   Your score from category A relates to your preference for interpersonal skills; category B reflects your mechanical/technical skills; and category C reflects skills and interests in data. This method of grouping skills adapts to nursing Holland's (1973) categories of people and environment. People skills include instructing or serving (statements 1, 2, 6, 7, and 8) and leading or managing (statements 3, 4, and 5) and are closely correlated with social and enterprising themes. Mechanical and technical skills center on things (statements 9, 10, 11, and 12) and correlate with a realistic interest theme. Data-oriented skills are either numerical (statements 13, 14, and 15), artistic (statements 17 and 18), or abstract statements (16, 19, 20, and 21) in emphasis and are similar to investigative, artistic, and conventional interest themes. Make comparisons. If there are dissimilar findings, ask yourself what that might mean in terms of actual experiences or perceptions of your skills.

Case Example B: Sample Profile of Attributes

In Exercise 5–8 you will summarize your attributes profile. This case example gives you an idea of how one nurse completed her profile.

Formal/informal education since completing requirements for RN licensure	Experiences and achievements (including years as RN)	Level of proficiency	Skills preference
Courses post-BSN: pathophysiology and holistic health	RN for 5 years: 2 yr staff nurse; 3 yr critical care	Proficient in nursing role related to drug trials	People; data
OJT clinical research with analgesics and anesthetics	Research Assistant to Anesthesiologist	Competent in critical care	
Self-taught advanced pharmacology, yoga, relaxation, and aerobics			

Exercise 5–8   Profile of Your Attributes

Referring to the results of your attributes assessment, complete the following with the appropriate information to summarize them.

Formal/informal education since completing requirements for RN licensure	Experiences and achievements (including years as RN)	Level of proficiency	Skills preferences
_____	_____	_____	_____
_____	_____	_____	_____
_____	_____	_____	_____
_____	_____	_____	_____

If asked, what would you say you like best about your personal attributes? Are they evident in your current career status? Answers to these questions are useful to you in determining where you are currently in your career, in establishing viable career goals, and in planning and managing your career.

Style

Your style is the expression of your essence as an individual; that memory of you etched in the minds of others. It is reflected in your verbal and nonverbal communication, in how you dress, in the priorities around which you focus your life, in how you learn, and in how you execute tasks. Your style radiates positive energy, ambivalence, lack of self-confidence, a zest for living, or the need to avoid risks and conform to rules. No doubt your style reflects themes that are the same as your interests and skills: realistic, artistic, conventional, enterprising, investigative, or social. Likewise, your style reflects your values. Three aspects of style are discussed here: lifestyle, learning style, and communication style. Looking at how you approach life, learning, and interacting with others leads to appreciation of the unique aspects of your style.

Lifestyle

Lifestyle is defined as the way three key ingredients work together, reinforcing one another in the ebb and flow of homeostatic balance: intellectual (mind), physical (body), and emotional (spirit) (Hagberg & Leider, 1982) (Figure 5–2). Although a sense of balance is optimum, an appreciation for individual pref-

Figure 5–2   Three key ingredients of lifestyle.

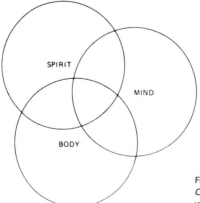

From Hagberg J, Leider R: *The Inventurers: Excursions in Life and Career Renewal*, p. 52. Reading, MA: Addison-Wesley, 1978, with permission.

erences in the interplay of these lifestyle components can be valuable in reflecting on prior career decisions and career management strategies.

Some common imbalances among mind, body and spirit are illustrated in Figures 5–3, 5–4, and 5–5. Those who tend to be guided more by feeling than by intellectual or physical activities place greater emphasis on the spirit component of the triad. Note the larger size of the spirit circle compared to the other two in Figure 5–3. Figure 5–4 illustrates a lifestyle configuration in which most emphasis is on physical activities (doing), the body component. A higher priority on intellectual pursuits or academic prowess is illustrated by a larger mind (knowing) circle in Figure 5–5.

Figure 5–3 Spirit (being) lifestyle influence.

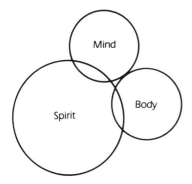

From Hagberg J, Leider R: *The Inventurers: Excursions in Life and Career Renewal,* p. 54. Reading, MA: Addison-Wesley, 1978, with permission.

Figure 5–4 Body (doing) lifestyle emphasis.

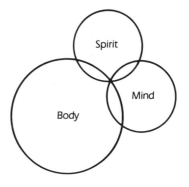

From Hagberg J, Leider R: *The Inventurers: Excursions in Life and Career Renewal,* p. 54. Reading, MA: Addison-Wesley, 1978, with permission.

Figure 5–5 Mind (knowing) lifestyle emphasis.

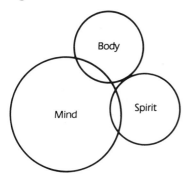

From Hagberg J, Leider R: *The Inventurers: Excursions in Life and Career Renewal,* p. 54. Reading, MA: Addison-Wesley, 1978, with permission.

Among the benefits of looking at the extent of balance or imbalance in your lifestyle triad as it applies to managing your nursing career is to match nursing setting, clients, focus, and function with your lifestyle. For example, if you place a higher emphasis on physical activities, you may prefer to focus on illness prevention and health promotion rather than on critical care or trauma care. Your lifestyle may support your choice of career goals or your satisfaction with where you are currently in your career.

In Exercise 5–9 nine qualities that reflect style have been selected. The results will help you construct a diagram of the interrelationships of the three lifestyle components in your life.

Exercise 5–9   Rating Individual Qualities That Reflect Your Style

Rate yourself on the quartile scale (series of four groups with equal frequency) for each item listed, indicating the extent to which you believe you possess these qualities.

Qualities		25%	50%	75%	100%
1. Creativity	♡				
2. Positive self-image	⚤				
3. Physical strength	⚤				
4. Intelligence	○				
5. Intuition	♡				
6. Physical energy	⚤				
7. Self-knowledge	○				
8. Spiritual strength	♡				
9. Wisdom	○				

Scoring

Use the following steps and scoring to calculate ratings for each lifestyle category.

Step 1: Enter the rating for each item in the appropriate space in the three categories.

Step 2: Add your ratings for each category of items, then divide the total by 3 to obtain your score.

A. ♡ Spirit

Item:· 1   5   8

Rating: _____

Your total score = _____ ÷ 3 = _____

B. ⚲ Body

Item: 2   3   6

Rating:_____

Your total score = _____ ÷ 3 = _____

C. ○ Mind

Item: 4   7   9

Rating: _____   Your total score = _____ ÷ 3 = _____

Use your score in each category as a guide for drawing three intertwined spirit, body, and mind circles in the space provided.

Your interpretation of the implications of your lifestyle on your career goals and the effect of your goals on your lifestyle will help you rank your preferred nursing options and formulate and weigh your career goals. It will also provide you with inspiration for using self-advocacy as a career management strategy. Lifestyle relating to career planning and management strategies is discussed in Chapters 8 and 9.

Learning Style

Learning styles are individual preferences for content, conditions, modes, activities, and situations related to the quest for knowledge. Like skills and interests, content preferences reflect an affinity for subjects related to data, people, or things. Individual preferences for learning conditions vary from teacher directed to self-directed and include factors such as focus on organization, detail, peer affiliation, competition, goal setting, and instructor affiliation. Canfield (1977) organizes learning modes into four activities: reading, doing, viewing, and listening. Kolb (1976) designed a learning style inventory as a self-description test based on experiential learning theory. According to Kolb (1976):

> Experiential learning is conceived as a four-stage cycle: (1) immediate concrete experience is the basis for (2) observation and reflection; (3) these observations are assimilated into a "theory" from which new implications for action can be deduced; (4) these implications or hypotheses then serve as guides in acting to create new experiences. The effective learner relies on four different learning modes: concrete experience, reflective observation, abstract conceptualization and active experimentation.

Using this method of learning, you would be able to involve yourself fully, openly, and without bias in new experiences, deliberate on and observe these experiences from many perspectives, create concepts that integrate your observations into logically sound theories, and apply these theories in making decisions and solving problems.

Kolb's four-stage cycle for experiential learning closely correlates with the problem-solving process illustrated in the career management framework. For example, immediate concrete experience is a prime source of information in the data-gathering phase as it relates to two of the three components (self and nursing) of the framework. Assessment of your immediate concrete nursing experience is your perceived level of proficiency (Exercise 5–6). Assessment of your life experiences, reflected in your lifestyle emphasis, is an example of how assessment of yourself fits this experiential model; assessment of your career stage corresponds to an experiential approach in assessing where you are now in your nursing career. Because of their futuristic emphasis, trends are incompatible with this first stage of an experiential approach. However, the context, in which you use your hypotheses as guides in creating new experiences, depends on a knowledge of trends as they relate to each of your hypothesized directions. Steps two and three of an experiential approach are specified components of the planning phase of problem solving. Effective planning requires observing and considering collected data as well as assimilating the results of this process into a theory or supposition from which new implications can be determined. From these implications, you can develop hypotheses to use as guides in translating your personal and professional goals into career goals and subsequent career management strategies.

According to Hagberg and Leider (1982) and as noted in Table 5–6, if you learn best through activities that involve *feeling,* you probably approach learn-

Table 5–6   Examples of Approaches to Learning

Feeling

Enthusiastic Involves and inspires other people Searches, seeks out new experiences Likes risks, excitement, change, incentives, and experiences	Imaginative Creates with emotions; aesthetic interest Imagines self in different situations Learns by listening, then sharing ideas with small number of people, or by modeling
Practical Applies ideas to solving problems Uses reason, logic to meet goals, take action Learns by looking at probabilities and testing them out, coming to conclusions	Logical Put ideas together to form a new model Uses precision and organization Learns by individually thinking through ideas and designing a plan or model in an organized way

Doing — Watching

Thinking

Adapted with permission from Hagberg J, Leider R: *The Inventurers: Excursions in Life and Career Renewal.* Reading, MA: Addison—Wesley, 1982.

ing enthusiastically and imaginatively; if you learn best by *watching,* you probably identify with both imaginative and logical approaches to learning; if you prefer learning situations requiring enthusiastic and practical approaches, you probably favor learning by *doing;* and if you use practical and logical approaches to learning, you presumably learn best from activities that require *thinking.*

The Hagberg and Leider categories of approaches to learning correlate closely with lifestyle emphases. They use four slightly different descriptions of learning styles and relate them to feeling, doing, thinking, and watching activities. They categorize learning styles as "enthusiastic, imaginative, practical, and logical." See Table 5–6 for examples. Thinking is closely related to a lifestyle emphasis on knowing (mind) and a predilection for gathering career-related information by reading. Watching activities are compatible with gathering information via observation. Doing clearly correlates with active experimentation as a data-gathering approach. With a feeling orientation and a being, or spirit, lifestyle emphasis, information gathering and career planning are likely to be approached using methods that involve feeling. No matter which style you prefer, all are congruent with a self-directed approach to managing your career in nursing. Self-assessment is the key to identifying and ranking your data gathering, career planning, and career management strategies.

Exercise 5–10 Learning Style Preference

Following is a list of 5 components related to learning style preference, learning situations, and learning approaches. Rank them within each category beginning with number 1, from most preferred to least preferred.

1. Content related to

   a. Words or language _____

   b. Numbers _____

   c. Things _____

   d. People _____

2. Learning by

   a. Reading _____

   b. Doing _____

   c. Viewing _____

   d. Listening _____

3. Learning conditions that are

   a. Organized _____

   b. Competitive _____

   c. Independent _____

   d. Participated in with others _____

   e. Directed by an instructor _____

   f. Focused on detail _____

4. Learning situations that involve

   a. Feeling _____

   b. Watching _____

   c. Doing _____

   d. Thinking _____

   e. Full and open involvement in new experiences _____

   f. Observation and reflection _____

   g. Abstract conceptualization _____

   h. Active experimentation _____

5. Learning approaches that are

   a. Enthusiastic _____

   b. Practical _____

   c. Imaginative _____

   d. Logical _____

Review your responses and write a description of your learning style in the space provided.

_____

_____

_____

A balance in approaches to learning enhances your flexibility in the selection of appropriate modes and conditions according to the content and situation, especially in formal teaching–learning environments. Awareness of your preferences and their congruence with your interests, skills, and lifestyle enables you to select optimum approaches to the self-directed pursuit of managing your nursing career.

Communication Style

The components of communication style cannot be overemphasized as a manifestation of your individual style. Body movements, facial expressions, silence, eye movement, eye contact, hand movements, handshake, stance, walk, voice tone and quality, smiling, frowning, sitting, touching, and movement toward or away from those with whom you are communicating are examples of frequently used nonverbal communication styles. Feedback, active listening, questioning, clarifying, restating, reflecting and clarifying, and using humor are examples of oral communication techniques. The specificity of the message, timing, and setting also are important in effective communication.

Exercise 5–11   Nonverbal Communication Style

What is your nonverbal communication style? For each of the following expressions, write a word or short phrase that best describes you. For feedback purposes, validating that your perception of your communication style is congruent with the perception of others, ask a friend, colleague, or family member to discuss this exercise with you.

Nonverbal communication	Description of self	Other's validation
1. Body movements	_____	_____
2. Facial expression	_____	_____
3. Silence	_____	_____
4. Eye movement	_____	_____
5. Eye contact	_____	_____
6. Hand movements	_____	_____
7. Handshake	_____	_____
8. Stance	_____	_____
9. Walk	_____	_____
10. Voice tone	_____	_____
11. Voice quality	_____	_____
12. Smiling	_____	_____
13. Frowning	_____	_____

Nonverbal communication	*Description of self*	*Other's validation*
14. Sitting	_____	_____
15. Touching	_____	_____
16. Position in relation to person with whom you are communicating	_____	_____

Exercise 5–12   Verbal Communication Style

Indicate with a check mark how often you use the following verbal strategies. Ask a friend, colleague, or family member to place a plus (+), indicating agreement, or a minus (−), indicating disagreement.

Verbal communication	Self-assessement of occurrence			Other's assessment
	Always	Usually	Rarely	(+/−)
1. Questioning				
2. Giving feedback				
3. Active listening				
4. Restating				
5. Reflecting				
6. Clarifying				
7. Using humor				
8. Giving advice				
9. Interrupting others				
10. Initiating comments				
11. Summarizing				
12. Stating feelings to others				
13. Accepting feedback				
14. Getting others to express feelings				
15. Getting others to express ideas				
16. Monopolizing the conversation				

Is your assessment of your communication style congruent with that of the person who assessed your responses? Communication requires a sender and a receiver; feedback is the key to the receiver's interpretation of your message. Asking for feedback from those with whom you communicate helps you evaluate the clarity of your own communication and the perceptions of others who receive it.

Your communication style strongly affects your career planning and management strategies. Your career progression is dependent on how clearly you communicate your career goals and actions. For example, if your nonverbal communication is assertive as communicated by eye contact, stance, or tone of voice and your verbal communication style is questioning to gain information, your message may be interpreted as overly aggressive. Your intention to negotiate may thus be interpreted as an intent to intimidate. Receiving messages from others that are inconsistent with the response you expected is cause to reexamine your communication style.

Nonverbal communication has a greater influence on your message than any possible array of words. Of course, communication is most effective when nonverbal and verbal messages are congruent. Some specific communication strategies for effective negotiating, marketing, and networking are discussed in Chapter 9. The following are general effective communication strategies:

1. Place yourself physically on the same level as the person with whom you are communicating.

2. Be sensitive to others' personal space in determining mutual comfort in proximity, distance, or touching.

3. Use an open posture (sitting relaxed, arms uncrossed, and an open facial expression) when seeking information.

4. Observe for nonverbal cues that your message is clear or confusing.

5. Listening astutely to verbal cues that corroborate the intent of your message or express that it is not clear.

6. Ask for feedback regarding clarity (for example, "Can I clarify that further?" "Do you understand what I'm saying/asking?") or use an open-ended approach (for example, "I'm wondering if I should restate . . . .").

7. Ask others for their verbal response to your message (for example, "So what do you think about my . . .?" "I'm interested in your response to . . . ." "Would you share with me your thoughts about . . . .").

This review of communication style and effective communication strategies will help you assess some aspects of your communication techniques and how you might apply them in developing your career goal.

Summary of Style

How would you describe your lifestyle, learning style, and communication style? In Exercise 5–13 think of words and phrases most descriptive of your style in these three areas. This summary and the summaries of personal characteristics, attributes, and stage, which you will complete subsequently, will be used to construct your profile.

Exercise 5–13 Summary of Your Style

Write words or short phrases that best summarize your style in the appropriate column.

Description of lifestyle	Description of learning style	Description of communication style

Stage

In Table 2–2 in Chapter 2, adult developmental stages were presented to help you establish your benchmark in terms of the interplay between your age, central purpose, and pervasive themes. Understanding adult developmental stages allows you to view your development in relation to other adults, and it is imperative that you consider these stages with openness and sensitivity. Rarely will others' themes and purposes exactly mirror yours. As with the developmental stages of children and adolescents, adult developmental stages often overlap and may be experienced in differing orders not necessarily associated with chronologic age. Furthermore, adult developmental stages often are more related to life events than to chronologic age. Pervasive themes and central life purposes affect career development. Effective career management is greatly enhanced by assessing consistencies and inconsistencies of your pervasive themes and central life purposes with your career stage.

Table 5–7 is an adaptation of adult development concepts with the addition of nurses' career stages. This table provides an opportunity to evaluate each of these concepts and stages. It enables you to reflect on the results in terms of career planning and management strategies. Read them with an attitude of exploration, searching for clues that seem to fit you. Use the first benchmark to record your results from Table 2–2 and the second to indicate with a check mark the nursing career stages that correspond most closely with where you are now in your nursing career.

Table 5–7   Adult Developmental Stages and Nurses' Career Stages

Age	Phase	Central Purposes and Pervasive Themes	Your Benchmark	Nurses' Career Stages	Your Benchmark
18–22	Transition to adulthood	*Exploring:* intimacy, independence, identity, involvement and ideals Wondering what you should do		Preparation via work experiences and or education Making first choices about career path	
23–30	Young adulthood	*Experiencing:* involvement with intimates, self-sufficiency, self-identity, and commitment to ideals Doing what you should do		Exploration and trial First position as an R.N. Early transfers and promotions Pursuing further education Developing an image of working as an R.N.	
30–37	Adulthood	*Settling:* Assuming responsibility for intimacy, identity, involvement, and ideals Juggling roles and responsibilities Knowing what you should do and wondering if you can		Establishment and advancement Reaffirmation of career choice Recommitment to nursing Orderly promotion, having a mentor Specializing, managing	
38–45	Transition to mid-adulthood	*Stabilizing:* Reviewing and revising previous decisions Openness to alternatives Exerting and asserting yourself Thinking what you could do, and doing it		Mid-career transitions Beginning a second career Changing career direction Expanding career horizons Consulting, leading, publishing	
46–53	Mid-adulthood	*Realization:* Balancing your life Renewed stability and vitality Enjoying self-confidence and security Doing what you know you can do		Career maintenance Contentment with being at the top of the pay scale Enjoying career accomplishments Balancing involvement in nursing career	
54–61	Transition to later adulthood	*Actualization:* Changing your sense of self and others Integrating yourself with your life choices Being, doing and enjoying it		Career role transitions Role modeling, coaching, and mentoring other nurses	
62–69	Later adulthood	*Deceleration:* Exploring alternatives Viewing life horizons Modeling ideals and values Doing what you like and liking what you do		Retirement or reduction in career involvement Disengagement from nursing career	
70–	Senior adulthood	*Reflection:* Self approval Doing what you are able to Remembering what you did		Career reflections	

Exercise 5–14 Summary Profile: Adult Developmental Stage and Nursing Career Stage

In the following columns record the information that best summarizes the central purpose and pervasive theme of your adult developmental and nursing career stages.

Your age range	Central purpose and pervasive theme	Nursing career stage
_____	_____	_____
	_____	_____

Since adult developmental stages tend to define your central life purpose and are pervasive themes that have an impact on your whole life, they affect and are affected by your career path. Awareness of where you are and of your characteristics, attributes, and style will help you complete your self-profile at the end of this chapter.

Are your central purposes and themes analogous to your nursing career stages? Or are you 35 years old and just now experiencing your first position as a registered nurse? Because of the diverse age range of nurses beginning their careers, it would not be unusual to find yourself juggling adult roles and responsibilities while in the preparatory or exploration and trial stage of your nursing career. Knowing where you are in terms of stage will help you devise a plan of where you want to be and by when.

Using Information About You

This chapter has helped you recognize that you are your own greatest resource and best advocate. From a variety of self-assessment exercises, you have collected and compiled information about personal and career characteristics important to you. This self-perspective is a substantial base on which to build your analysis of nursing options and match your profile with preferred options. You will also find yourself referring to the results of specific self-assessment exercises as you design your career plan and use effective strategies for managing your career.

Your Personal Profile

Your personal profile is a combination of your characteristics, attributes, style, personal developmental stage, and career stage, which identifies you as an individual. Exercise 5–15 will help you summarize this kaleidoscopic image of yourself for use in a comprehensive exercise at the end of Chapter 6, where you will match your profile with selected nursing options. Additionally, as you develop your career plan and explore strategies for effective career management, you will again refer to this compilation of highly significant information about you.

Your profile also helps you formulate a personal goal. Your goal is a statement of what you *really* want to be doing and for what reasons. It reflects the outcomes or rewards you seek in your life. This goal projects what you want to achieve in roughly 3 to 5 years.

Your goal should reflect your characteristics, attributes, style, and stage. The more closely you align these features with career goals, the easier it will be for you to manage your career satisfactorily. Keep your profile and goals in focus as you explore the range of nursing options. You will integrate this information about yourself with information about nursing in Chapter 6. The following case example demonstrates use of information about personal characteristics, attributes, style and stage in the formulation of a personal goal.

Case Example: Sharon

Sharon values self-growth and spirituality. She listed meaningful work and continual self-development among her five most important needs. Her dominant interest themes are investigative and social. She completed a baccalaureate nursing program 5 years ago and has worked in critical care ever since. Sharon assessed her level of proficiency as expert and her skills preferences as people and data. Her lifestyle emphasizes mind and spirit; she learns best by reading and logical approaches. Active listening dominates her communication style. Sharon, age 26, is single and is in the process of establishing and advancing her nursing career. She stated one of her goals as follows: "I want to be involved with meaningful work in a place where I can continue to learn both formally and informally."

Exercise 5–15 *Summarizing Your Profile and Identifying Your Personal Goals*

Review exercises 5–4, 5–8, 5–13, and 5–14. As you do so, think of the most significant words or short phrases that best describe your characteristics, attributes, stage, and style. Record them in the appropriate columns that follow. Using these features formulate a personal goal statement.

Characteristics	Attributes	Stage	Style

Goal: _____

_____

_____

References

Benner P: *From Novice to Expert,* pp. 20–36. Menlo Park, CA: Addison-Wesley, 1984.

Bolles RN: *What Color is Your Parachute?* Berkeley: Ten Speed Press, 1986.

Canfield A: *Learning Styles Inventory.* Plymouth, MI: Humanics Inc., 1977.

Hagberg J, Leider R: *The Inventurers: Excursions in Life and Career Renewal,* pp. 36; 53–55; 82–83. Reading, MA: Addison-Wesley, 1982.

Holland J: *Making Vocational Choices—A Theory of Careers.* New York: Prentice-Hall, 1973.

Johansson C: *Career Assessment Inventory Profile.* Minneapolis, MN: National Computer Systems, 1980.

Kolb D: *Learning Style Inventory,* p. 3. Boston: McBer and Co, 1976.

6 Assessing the Options

BARBARA O. McGETTIGAN

The labels nurse, teacher, manager come to mind when we think of nursing options. Although these are appropriate and useful ways to identify nursing, they only begin to describe the breadth of nursing practice. The labels refer to roles but do not address other key aspects of nursing practice such as setting, client, or focus. What characteristics or dimensions, then, are helpful for full exploration of the scope of practice options? How can you use these dimensions to construct several possible directions for nursing goals?

This chapter explores selected dimensions of nursing practice. With each, you will have an opportunity for analysis and self-appraisal. After a full analysis, you will design several options. These are professional goals that reflect your personal characteristics, attributes, style, and stage as well as your interests and preferences for nursing practice. These goals define, clarify or confirm what you want to do in your nursing career. When considering your options, be as explorative and unrestrained as possible so you will be most creative. Your creative thinking is balanced in Chapter 7 with realism that evolves from considering trends and future projections.

Professional Dimensions

Analyzing nursing options can be confusing and sometimes frustrating because of inconsistencies and ambiguities in terminology. Words like *independent practice* and *practitioner* or *clinical specialist, clinician,* and *clinical nurse specialist* are used interchangeably in the literature and in the practice arena—terms overlap. We describe nursing practice in general terms but use a specific label, practitioner, to refer to a special group of nurses with refined, advanced assessment, and client management skills. We refer to specializing with little general agreement on requirements. Williamson (1983) reflects on these dilemmas of terminology as seemingly "symptomatic of our failure to reach consensus regarding the structure of our discipline."

As the nursing profession evolves, theory builds, and society expects greater professional accountability, the semantic problem should resolve. In the interim, however, you should develop a terminology and an approach for analyzing nursing practice to develop nursing options. Without definitions or a structure, analyzing and exploring nursing options becomes, at best, unwieldy. With a structure, you can conduct a more comprehensive analysis of practice, broaden your perspective of options, and increase your ability to tailor your nursing practice to you.

Designing a nursing structure involves asking how many nursing dimensions there are and how these can combine to express your practice. The major components within nursing knowledge are client, environment or setting, nursing, and health (Fawcett, 1980; 1984). For the purpose of presenting a method for analysis of nursing options in this chapter, the health component is divided into health problem and human response; the nursing component is viewed from both a function and a role perspective. In all, there are six components for your analysis of nursing practice: client, setting, health problem, human response, nursing functions, and roles.

Over the past 30 years, emphasis on these dimensions has changed. The 1950s and 1960s emphasized the nature of client–nurse interaction. This shifted in the 1960s and 1970s to the client per se and to the health problem and human response with the start of the 1980s. The future may reiterate the importance of the early emphasis on environment seen in Florence Nightingale's practice. The investigations and concerns of the nursing profession change and deepen with new understandings and theory applied to practice.

Each nurse as a professional seeks an area of emphasis for practice. This may change over time with the influence of professional or societal interests or with shifts in personal values, needs, and experiences. Figure 6–1 illustrates dimensions for analysis of nursing options. Considering these dimensions is essential for a thorough analysis of nursing practice. Only after a thorough examination can you begin to synthesize them into several different nursing options.

As a nurse, you can select and highlight certain aspects of each of these dimensions, combining them into a practice. The result is a personal career. The selections within each dimension are numerous, escalating in variety as all dimensions interact. Finally, much as the cube can be positioned to rest on any side, you can base your practice on any one dimension. For many nurses, the health problem is the foundation; for other nurses, client response or even a client group forms the foundation and ultimately supports the other aspects of practice.

Figure 6–1   *Dimensions for analysis of nursing options.*

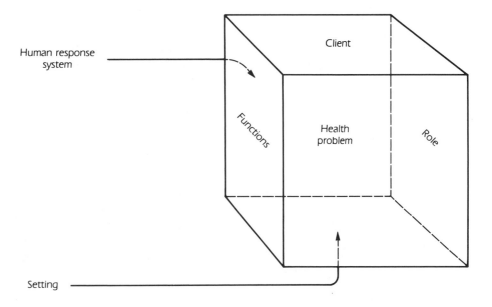

Requirements and Personal Considerations

In your analysis of nursing options, explore the requirements and suitability of your personal attributes and traits to various dimensions of practice. With this information, you can differentiate what simply might be of interest to you from what is right for you given your knowledge, skill, values, and needs or style and stage. Also, keeping requirements in mind helps you appraise current feasibility of career goals and make meaningful plans for the future.

Requirements

Requirements for dimensions of practice include academic degrees, special training, certificates, levels on career ladders, years of general or specialized experience, and demonstrated knowledge and skill. In nursing there are few clear stipulations about requirements for nursing options. Guidelines that have been developed are often unevenly implemented. Requirements for degrees, number of years, or type of experiences related to positions are often ambiguous. For instance, does a Bachelor of Science (BS) with a major in nursing or a BS in health systems management meet the degree requirement for the head nurse role? Does a Master of Science in nursing (MSN) or one in business administration (MBA) meet the requirements for nursing administration? Does a nursing home director need experience in a skilled nursing facility (SNF), or would hospital management experience be comparable? Does the staff nurse need 1 or 2 years of general nursing experience before specializing in one clinical area or before moving into home health nursing? How can you decipher these requirements? Where can you turn?

To deal with ambiguities in requirements, consider what is actually needed to perform the tasks involved in the option. This assessment of knowledge, skill, or attitudes related to performance is the most practical and useful way to delineate requirements. If you are exploring a nursing administrative role, assess the functions involved and judge the knowledge and skills that will be required for that option. If you are exploring an executive role in a nursing home, special knowledge and skill related to long-term care would be an additional requirement for that option. If you are focusing on interpersonal problems, you need to analyze special communication knowledge and skills. As you reflect on the various nursing dimensions such as role, setting, or focus, ask yourself what basic and essential background is required.

In addition to requirements directly related to specific tasks of practice, some requisites are less obviously linked to performance, including those established by legislation or regulations, recommended by professional or accrediting agencies, and followed as common practice within an area. These requirements might be degrees, certificates, or years of experience in a field or specialty.

Legislation and regulatory agencies stipulate minimum requirements to protect the public. State departments of health or boards of nursing regulate minimum requirements for positions in some types of settings, in basic nursing programs, and in some overlapping or independent roles such as nurse practitioner or midwife. It is essential to identify the regulatory agencies involved in the options you are considering.

Organizations such as The Joint Commission for Accreditation of Hospitals or the National League for Nursing recommend guidelines that often imply requirements for certain positions. An agency that seeks accreditation follows these requirements to a great extent. Ascertaining organizations involved in accrediting a particular practice setting is also very important in assessing requirements.

Professional organizations such as the American Nurses' Association establish standards for practice and certification for education beyond minimum safety. They indicate what is optimal to insure quality outcomes of nursing service. Organizations involved in certification play a significant role in establishing and maintaining requirements for recognition of professional levels with a specialty focus.

The extent that institutions implement requirements related to professional or accrediting agencies varies with the economy and numbers in the work force. Availability of money and people to meet various requirements sets a level of expectation and common practice in an area as well as in the entire country. Thus, it is important to track national and state statistics. For example,

Table 6–1 shows the 1980 national norms for the highest educational preparation related to nursing titles.

Although confusing or at times frustrating, variability in requirements can provide you with latitude. Given negotiation and self-advocacy skills, you may demonstrate expertise and position-relevant skills attained from comparable experiences and/or education. Negotiating on requirements, however, implies an honest appraisal of what is needed and of your personal level of knowledge and skill.

For instance, you may be interested in a management role but not have the required years of experience or the required degree. The skills you have gained from 10 years of volunteer work for a nurses' association in budgets, program planning, personnel selection, and evaluation may compare to the tasks described in the role. With creative and honest appraisal, you can show that these skills meet the job requirements.

Perhaps you are interested in a clinical nurse specialist role that demands an MSN. Since you have been active nationally in establishing a specialty organization and its standards for care, you are aware that many who fill such

TABLE 6–1   Distribution of Registered Nurses Among Positions in Nursing Service Management, Nurse Education, and Clinical Specialties by Highest Educational Preparation, November 1980

Title	Total	Associate Degree	Diploma	Baccalaureate	Masters	Doctorate
Administrator or assistant	100	9.7	46.7	24.0	18.2	1.4
Consultant	100	8.8	39.3	28.2	23.2	0.5
Supervisor or assistant	100	17.4	59.8	19.4	3.4	—
Instructor (all nurse educators)	100	7.0	20.1	32.2	38.2	2.5
Nurse practitioner midwife	100	10.5	40.1	30.1	19.1	0.2
Clinical nurse specialist	100	15.3	36.7	20.2	27.1	0.7
Nurse clinician	100	14.0	43.9	26.8	13.0	2.3
Nurse anesthetist	100	19.5	55.5	23.4	1.6	—
Totals	100	20.2	51.1	23.4	5.1	0.2

From the Department of Health and Human Services, Health Resources Administration: The Registered Nurse Population, an Overview. National Sample Survey of Registered Nurses, Nov. 1980 (Report 82–5, revised June 1982). Hyattsville, MD.

roles in your area do not hold Master degrees. Comparable experiences may be adequate to meet the requirements in this case.

In many situations requirements are negotiable. Legal requirements are usually more rigid than organizational ones, although some exceptions are made on appeal for special circumstances. Assess well the intent of requisites, their source, and the degree of interpretation possible. Appraise yourself according to the knowledge and skills needed for options. Decide if gaps can be bridged, if you want to bridge them, and how you plan to do so.

Personal Considerations

Personal considerations such as your needs, values, style, and stage may be more consistent with some practice dimensions than with others. When personal factors are addressed, your work certainly rewards you either extrinsically or intrinsically. Some nurses need external, tangible rewards such as a comfortable work space, a title, promotion opportunities, or a raise in salary. Others need or want intrinsic rewards from decision-making opportunities, available resources, or respect from co-workers. Whatever the needs or values, consider practice from the perspective of these very personal dimensions. For example, if you seek high self-esteem or power, consider practice in a critical care or hemodialysis unit, where physician–nurse collaboration, status among nurses, and a pay differential could meet these needs. If you need independence and autonomy, you might favor primary nursing in an agency or explore consulting or independent business options.

Salary varies tremendously by geography, by setting, and even by individuals within the same setting. Salary differences stem from availability of people and money and from negotiation skills of individual nurses or bargaining units. Table 6–2 gives a sampling of 1982 salaries. Obvious differences among roles must be appreciated. The person considering an instructor role should recognize the relatively low salary of faculty compared to that for nursing administration or management in a hospital.

Applying personal style and stage to nursing also gives you a clearer picture of suitable options. Reflecting on mind, body, and spirit components in various nursing dimensions helps you appreciate subtle and intangible features of practice. For instance, physical demands on a general unit staff nurse contrast with technical, detailed approaches of the nurse in a neonatal intensive care unit (NICU). A nurse with high-stress tolerance who thrives in a fast-paced setting seems suited to critical care, but the person who prefers mental, methodical work might consider quality assurance more consistent with style.

Stage in life should be considered with options. A nursing faculty member at the establishment stage might seek a progressive, challenging new program, whereas this nurse at a later stage might find the stability of a long-established school more appealing. A novice would seek opportunities for skill develop-

TABLE 6–2   Estimated Average Salaries of Full-time Registered Nurses by Employment Setting and Position

Employment Setting and Position	Actual November 1980	Estimated January 1982	Estimated Average Annual Percentage Increase
Average			
All full-time registered nurses	$17,393	$19,381	9.8
Hospital			
Administrative	24,620	27,865	11.3
Supervisor	19,820	22,387	11.1
Clinical nursing specialist	19,412	21,609	9.7
Nurse clinician	19,675	22,062	10.4
Head nurse	17,719	19,600	9.1
Staff nurse	16,451	18,331	9.8
Nursing home			
Administrative	17,304	18,676	6.8
Staff nurse	14,332	16,020	10.1
Nursing education			
Instructor	18,766	21,022	10.3
Public health			
Administrative	20,829	23,672	11.7
Supervisor	17,961	19,637	8.0
Staff nurse	15,068	16,334	7.2
Student health			
Staff nurse	14,578	16,040	8.5
Occupational health			
Staff nurse	18,710	21,155	11.2
Physician's office			
Staff nurse	11,938	12,872	6.7
Nurse practitioner/midwife			
All settings	19,395	21,726	10.3

November 1980 data: from Levine E, Moses EB: A Statistical profile of registered nurses in the United States 1977–1980. USDHHS, DHPA Report No. 82–3, p. 21.
Estimated average annual percentage increases: from Levine E, Moses EB: A statistical profile of registered nurses in the United States 1977–1980. USDHHS, DHPA Report No. 82-3, p. 21. (adjusted to reflect the fact that the period September 1977–November 1980 is 38 months, not 3 years).
January 1982 estimates: extrapolated from November 1980 data for the 14-month interval.

ment, but the expert would seek ways to use knowledge and skills in fulfilling and challenging work.

As you read descriptions of dimensions of nursing practice, judge your interests and preferences. Keep in mind your knowledge about self. Ask not only whether the options seem important and interesting to you, but whether you meet or want to meet requirements and can anticipate rewards significant to you.

Client

The client is the dimension of nursing that your practice serves. The client may be an individual or a specific group. In exploring clients as individuals, identify the traits, stage, and style of persons with whom you prefer to practice. For example, in considering stage are you captured by the physical development of the young, the social complexities of the middle-aged, or the psychologic adjustments of the elderly? Does the mature person who is suddenly struck by a heart attack draw your empathy, or does the distrustful adolescent who attempts suicide evoke your healing sensitivities? Are there style dimensions that you prefer? Is it the fast-track business person or the traditional homemaker who draws your nursing interventions? Consider racial, sexual, and cultural factors and the degree of diversity or congruence with your background and interests. Were you raised in a minority culture but now seek the challenge of dealing with diverse clients in metropolitan centers? Do you prefer to work with women as they deal with social change? Are you drawn to migrant farmers whose experiences and lifestyles are of major concern to your community?

Also think of clients in terms of groups, which are formed by family relationships, by shared health problems, or by other dimensions such as age or geography. Examples of options relating to client groups include the nurse teaching classes for diabetics in a health maintenance organization and the nurse performing cardiac rehabilitation work with groups clustered by specific diseases. School nurses may define clients as all children enrolled in district schools. For others, children at risk for hypertension or obesity may be the client groups.

A community is the client for some nurses. For instance, a nurse consultant for a city mental health advisory board serves the whole city population. For nurses in some state and national organizations and those working in other health-related organizations or regulatory agencies, the client is the whole nursing profession. For nurse educators, the client is groups of students.

You can see that nurses perceive clients differently. The better you delineate the client dimension of practice, the better you develop career options. If your interest and style calls for working with individual clients, maintain that facet of your practice. If you want to devote high energy and prefer working with large groups, design your career options with those personal characteristics in mind.

Exercise 6–1 Client Preference

Complete the following statements by writing your description of client.

1. I find that I work best with clients who have the following personal traits:

———————————————————————————————

———————————————————————————————

2. Clients in this stage of life:

   _____

   _____

3. Clients with this lifestyle:

   _____

   _____

4. Clients with this education or experiential background:

   _____

   _____

5. I work more effectively with clients in these groupings (specify individuals, small groups, organizations as a whole, or other):

   _____

   _____

   _____

   _____

6. How do preferred client characteristics or groupings relate to *your* stage, style, characteristics, and attributes?

   _____

   _____

   _____

The Setting

Nursing is practiced in a variety of settings, and that variety continues to expand. When picturing nursing practice, the hospital setting often comes first to mind. There is some accuracy in that image, since approximately three of every four nurses work in hospitals or nursing homes. Table 6–3 compares the numbers and percentage of nurses by various settings.

Table 6–4 presents changes by setting from 1977 to 1980. Certainly increases have been greatest in hospitals and nursing homes, but growth in nursing education and occupational health are also apparent. The diagnosis-related group (DRG) payment system is forcing the delivery of many more services in ambulatory settings such as surgicenters, doctors' offices, and outpatient departments of hospitals. Coleman and associates (1984) project that ambulatory

TABLE 6–3 Estimated Percentage of Nurses by Employment Setting

Employment Setting	Estimated Percentage
Hospital	65.6
Nursing home or extended-care facility	8.0
Public/community health (includes state, city, and county health departments, visiting nurse associations, community mental health centers, family planning centers, well-baby clinics, and combination nursing services)	6.5
Physicians' or dentists' office (includes solo, partnership, and group practices as well as health maintenance organizations)	5.7
Student health service (includes public and private elementary and secondary schools and colleges or universities)	3.5
Nursing education (includes all levels of nursing education)	3.6
Occupational health (government and private industry)	2.3
Private duty nursing	1.6
Self-employed	0.9
Other	1.7
Not known	0.6

Nurses today: A statistical portrait. *AJN* 1982; 82:450.

TABLE 6–4 Employed Registered Nurses by Work Setting, 1977 and 1980

Work Setting	Number Employed		1977–1980 Change	
	1977*	1980†	Number	(%)
Hospital	601,011	835,647	234,636	39.0
Nursing home	79,647	101,209	21,562	27.1
Public/community health	77,139	83,440	6301	8.2
Physician's/dentist's office	69,263	71,974	2711	3.9
Student health service	41,365	44,906	3541	8.6
Nursing education	37,826	46,504	8678	22.9
Occupational health	24,317	29,164	4847	19.9
Private duty	28,563	20,240	−8323	−29.1
Other and unknown	19,102	39,768	20,666	108.2
Total	978,234	1,272,851	294,617	30.1

*Figures from Roth A et al: *1977 National Sample Survey of Registered Nurses: A report on the nurse population and factors affecting their supply*, (NTIS Pub. HRP-0900603) Kansas City, MO, 1979, Table 51, p. 183.
†Figures from DHHS, HRA: The registered nurse population, an overview. In *National Sample Survey of Registered Nurses, November 1980*, (Report 82-5, revised June 1982) Hyattsville, MD, Table 5, p. 13.

Institute of Medicine: *Nursing and Nursing Education: Public Policy and Private Action*. Washington, DC: National Academy Press, 1983.

care will grow more than 200% in the next 3 years. Undoubtedly, increased ambulatory care decreases the number of nurses employed by hospitals, especially in nonintensive care units, and greatly increases the number of nurses in home care and health maintenance organizations. Careful analysis of setting becomes more and more important as the health care delivery system shifts from hospital to alternate settings.

The specific environment of a setting deserves careful analysis and a different emphasis than nurses have given it in the past. Often, in selecting sites the function directed the choice of setting. With growth and change in places and opportunities both in health-related and nonhealth agencies, you can select the characteristics of place that are important to satisfactory realization of nursing practice. The closer you match the philosophy, value, style, and expectations of a setting to your own, the greater your contentment and the more effective your practice in that setting. With a mismatch, place can restrict, confine, and dominate your practice.

Optimum person–environment fit takes careful analysis. From among the many and interrelated characteristics, four aspects of setting are important to assessment: degree of health relatedness, type of health care agency, organizational profile, and the self-employment option. When considering each of these aspects of setting, keep in mind your personal traits and how your values will or will not effectively interact with various types of settings.

Degree of Health Relatedness

Settings can be health agencies, health-related agencies, or nonhealth agencies. Some nurses are most comfortable in agencies directed solely toward health care. Health-related settings are typified by pharmaceutical companies, health supply companies, health or hospital associations, hospital management firms, and, of course, hospitals and nursing homes. Other nurses seek perspectives of a nonhealth-related setting. Examples are occupational nurses in industry, health counselors in colleges, flight nurses, cruise nurses, and nurses in senior centers, social service agencies, jails, or government agencies.

One nurse interested in self-care of handicapped persons chose to practice in a nonhealth-focused agency designing instructional software for robotics. This nurse valued a pioneering atmosphere and was drawn to technology. Another nurse, a nurse educator also interested in self-care, chose a rehabilitation hospital setting as consistent with meaningful clinical practice.

Type of Health Care Agency

Inpatient care institutions include hospitals and nursing homes. Ambulatory care settings include hospital outpatient departments, public health departments, doctors' offices, day care centers, specialty treatment centers, home care, and even mobile services to clients.

In assessing the match between you and these various health agencies, one factor to consider is the degree of client dependency. Inpatient care connotes clients receiving continuous monitoring, medical treatment, nursing treatment, and physical care. In ambulatory care settings, clients come and go and depend less on the nurse for physical care. The nurse in the inpatient environment often is compensating for the clients' inabilities to engage in self-care. Nursing actions and relationships differ in ambulatory care, where clients need ongoing support and education to overcome self-care limitations.

In addition to client dependency and self-care considerations, it is useful to reflect on length of client contact. Typically, the more acute and critical the setting; the shorter the duration of client contact. Considering these factors is helpful in choosing between inpatient care and ambulatory care settings. However, multiple factors interact, such as stage in life, economics, and availability of positions. For example, one nurse, a marathon runner with an interest in aerobics and sports medicine, found the hospital's sports clinic a most suitable setting. But, given a current life situation of caring for a young family, this same nurse found that a part-time position in a skilled nursing facility met current time and economic needs. In addition to style and personal characteristics, stage influences choice of health agency and setting.

Organizational Profile

In analyzing setting for employment, there are features such as size and services, structure, management and ownership, and culture that can be more or less suited to your personal goals and professional values or intents. Awareness of your preferences for these organizational features helps you explore and identify settings in which you want to work.

Size and Services. Consider whether you want to work in a large, small, urban, rural, research, or community hospital. Overall size and services run the gamut. Some large organizations such as Sloan Kettering Memorial Cancer Center in New York City have one specialty along with unit subspecialties (Malanka, 1984). Small community hospitals in rural or suburban areas may offer a broad range of client services. Your clinical background directs choice of type of agency somewhat. Personal style and values must also be consistent with level and type of services. Large, sophisticated tertiary care settings with changing technologies, research, and complex treatment modalities require nurses interested in new developments, in specializing, and in career advancement opportunities. By contrast, if you value a generalist perspective and see the role of the nurse as providing healing environments, you would find a community hospital more suitable for practice.

Structure. Size and structure often go hand-in-hand; the greater the number of people, tasks, and services, the more complex the organizational chart. Perhaps you are a person who wants a boss with direct and simple links to the board of directors. A home health agency, where the director of nursing reports to the board, might be the direct-line organization you seek. On the other hand, if you thrive on complex, multiple links, where power and policies challenge, you may find multihospital or multiservice corporations a more suitable structural profile. Some apparently small organizations are in fact very complex in structure. You may seek a hospital with a for-profit corporation, a foundation, and ambulatory services all separately incorporated yet administered by an umbrella corporate entity that provides support service to each of the subsidiary corporations. Thus, it is necessary to look closely at the complexity and type of structure that provide the optimum environment for you.

Management. Regardless of size, services, or structure, organizations manage work in diverse ways. Some are top–down and autocratic; others involve staff in a democratic process. You can assess the degree of autocracy and centralization and remoteness of control by deciphering how decisions are made, finding out who has the "last word," and identifying the membership on policy, practice, and hospital committees. Selected findings of the Magnet Study (McClure et al., 1983) and other reports of positive environmental characteristics within nursing departments (Muff, 1982; West, 1983; Malanka, 1984; Sovie, 1984) are listed in Table 6–5. Based on your personal and professional values and needs, environmental characteristics, such as the degree of power and participation by nurses in policy formulation and decision making, may be more or less key determinants in choosing a setting.

Ownership. Ownership relates much about who ultimately is in control. Is an agency a government or public facility, nonprofit such as university or religion-affiliated hospitals, or is it investor-owned and operated for profit? An organization's philosophy of care, management, and operational system often

Table 6–5   Positive Characteristics of Nursing Departments

1. Interdisciplinary practice committee with nursing, medical, and administrative membership
2. Parity of nursing and medical departments with direct accountability to hospital governing board
3. Primary broad-based nursing by professional nurses responsible for independent nursing care decisions and patient teaching, writing standards, and nurse-to-nurse consultation
4. Adequate staffing such as 1:1 RN to occupied bed, including administrative positions
5. Flexible work hours and patterns such as four 10-hour, five 8-hour, or three 12-hour shifts
6. Intellectual stimulation with opportunities for continuing education, specialty training, preceptorships, and tuition reimbursement
7. Decentralization with responsibility and decision making at the individual nursing unit level
8. Adequate salary and benefit packages
9. Career advancement and ladder opportunities in both clinical and management tracks
10. Visible and accessible director of nursing
11. Strong and accountable quality assurance program

reflect the type of ownership and control. With the growing number of university and public hospitals being purchased by the for-profit hospital or health care chains, issues of shareholder versus medical school or community board control are becoming increasingly sensitive (USNWR, 1984). Some people fear that when choices of resources have to be made, profit will take priority over quality in research, education, or service.

Awareness of these potential value conflicts will encourage you to analyze the ownership of a setting carefully. For instance, those who are inclined toward for-profit motives and a corporate model may fit more naturally into the proprietary or investor-owned rather than in the nonprofit or government-owned agency. Others with strong attitudes about the poor's access to medical care or a strong spiritual dimension in health care may prefer a nonprofit or religion-oriented agency.

Financing. In addition to ownership, how the health care services are financed is relevant to choice of setting. The nurse who values client access to a range of comprehensive services in exchange for a fixed prepayment fee might choose to work in health maintenance organizations (HMOs). The nurse who thinks that buyers, such as employers or unions, play a significant role in negotiating fees and seeking the most economic health care alternatives might select from among health care agencies that are part of preferred provider organizations (PPOs). All health care agencies are responding to limitations on reimbursements and exploring various ways to guarantee adequate numbers, or a "market share," of clients. It is helpful to consider subtle differences in arrangements. Compare those that attract clients with low fees by limiting services to those that emphasize reform and provide the most economic and appropriate alternatives for client care.

Climate. Ingalls (1976) suggests analyzing whether corporate climate is certainty oriented rather than ambiguity oriented. Rigid protocols, lots of "red tape," low risk taking, slow change, interpersonal conflict, and distrust reflect an environment with a high need for certainty. This contrasts with an atmosphere of creativity, informality, collaboration, and risk taking that indicates a tolerance for ambiguity. Matching your need for certainty or ambiguity with that found in an organization helps you ensure a better person–environment fit. Your tendencies and needs can conflict with those within an organization. Do you seek answers and certainty, or do you wrestle with problem identification and tolerate ambiguity?

Deal and associates (1983) find that corporate culture is recognized as "the way we do things around here." Culture specifies an agency's values and beliefs as seen in mottos or slogans, heroes, rituals such as meeting protocols and events, stories, and networks for communication. The culture defines the norms of behavior within a setting. If consistent and strong, culture results in better performance. If weak or in conflict, persons receive mixed messages, policies may dominate, and the organization is confused.

There can be optimum personality and culture matches. The person who likes competitive sports does well in a "macho" culture; the detailed, data-oriented person works most effectively within a "process" culture; and the social team player fits in well within the "work hard/play hard" culture. In assessing an organization's profile, it is helpful to consider culture, its strength, consistency, type, and suitability to you.

Self-Employment

Although nurses are often employed by others, opportunities for and interest in self-employment are on the rise. Nurse practitioners, midwives, expert clinicians, or specialists have established their own practices, many very successfully (Kinlein, 1977; Simms, 1977; Carr, 1982). In addition to private practice, nurses have started businesses as diverse as independent home care, publishing companies, continuing education and travel study businesses, nursing management or data process consulting for government and private health agencies (*Calif Nurse,* 1984). Establishing a private practice or a business enables nurses to combine unique interests and talents, express creativity, govern practice, and realize personal and professional goals. Self-employed nurses can achieve more flexibility, autonomy, and independence as well as potential financial gain. Disadvantages for nurses in business or private practice include 24-hour responsibility and limited third-party reimbursements that can threaten financial stability.

Starting a business or private practice requires much knowledge, skill, and certain characteristics. Professional level expertise in the service area is needed. Career experiences, including leadership roles, can pave the way for independent practice or business. You must be able to describe clearly services or products, set goals, and delineate targets or clients for services. For a clinical practice, a sound conceptual basis is essential. Establishing hospital privileges or developing business partnerships requires negotiation skills and knowledge of planned change. Professional know-how must be combined with awareness of the "territory": the community, its needs, clients, the health care agencies, and a network of influential nursing, medical, and hospital contacts.

The financial side of business includes establishing fees that are competitive but adequate to cover expenses and provide a reasonable profit. At least a rudimentary knowledge of business planning, marketing, reimbursement, and relevant laws and requirements is necessary. You need a great deal of time, especially at the start, and a willingness to take risks. You must also be able to handle a degree of isolation, fear of failure, and initial unstable income. But getting business referrals through networking and being visible provides a unique sense of accomplishment.

The importance of continuing this trend toward independent business is expressed well by Coleman and associates (1984):

> Unless nurses win policy-making priorities in the evolving systems or
> unless they develop their own revenue generating businesses strong

enough to contract with large holding corporations, they are unlikely to attain the control which managing finances brings.

Consider nurses who exemplify varied approaches to self-employment.

Case Example: Mary

Mary, a nurse educator expert at all nursing levels, contracted with area nursing schools to counsel potential applicants. For Mary, near retirement after a long career, the strong network to gain clients made this independent practice work.

Case Example: Lucy

Lucy, a registered nurse, had worked in nursing for 10 years and had saved a sizeable amount of money. To be successful as an independent professional, Lucy explored community trends and detected an unmet need. A new venture to meet that need was a health promotion program for senior retirement communities. In developing this business, Lucy drew on personal experiences but also hired geriatric nurse advisors. The business was incorporated and attracted venture capital, leading to expansion and a statewide business.

Both of these nurses were in different life and career stages, had different styles and values, yet were able to take risks, make commitments, build knowledge and skills related to their profession and to business in general, and work toward fulfillment or success. Both had adequate financial security to venture into a potentially insecure situation. Both relied on contacts developed through career, education, or volunteer work.

Having explored self-employment and selected features and types of work settings, take time now to reflect. In the following exercise, record your preferences and thoughts about the setting, a key dimension of your practice and a major facet of career options.

Exercise 6–2 Setting Considerations

Write your responses for each of the following considerations of setting.

1. Given a choice between a health agency or another type of setting, I prefer to work in the following (describe three possible settings):

   a. _____

   b. _____

   c. _____

2. I prefer an organization with the following profile (describe):

   a. A size of _____

      with services of _____

   b. A structure that is _____

      and management that is _____

   c. A _____ownership

   d. Climate or culture that is _____

      and _____financing

3. For me, self-employment is _____

Focus

In addition to client and setting, exploring the focus of your nursing practice unfolds a key dimension of practice and the major factor in developing nursing options. Nurses most commonly define their practice using the language of medicine, referring to themselves by medical interventions: medical nurse, surgical nurse, anesthesia nurse, enterostomal specialist, chemotherapeutic specialist. Williamson (1983) found that graduate programs in nursing described over 130 combinations of specific areas of study, many of which borrow from the medical model. Imitating medicine limits nursing. With the unique nursing context, however, nurses are guided in both research and practice. Given the stage of professional growth and theory building as well as the economic demands for reimbursement of specific services and cost containment, it is evident that nurses need to define clearly the specific and intended outcomes of their practice, using a nursing emphasis.

The ANA Social Policy statement (1980) interprets nursing as the diagnosis and treatment of human response to actual or potential health problems. The core or substance of nursing, however, is more than what nurses do, more than diagnosis and treatment. Nursing is more than the actual and potential health problems that are addressed. The concern and unique focus of nursing is assisting clients to cope effectively and to integrate biologic, psychologic, and/or social responses in an adaptive way. This focus is variously referred to as a person's adaptation, active management of self-care, client's self-regulation, and coping. Loomis and Wood (1983) aptly state that "the focus of the nurse's diagnosis and treatment is the patient's self-regulation of the human responses that interact with their health problems." Nursing's general focus and outcome of care is client coping or adjustment. Depending on the health problem and how it affects a person's life, nurses help clients deal with different experiences. Nurses have an opportunity and a need to focus their practice using specific problems as well as client response systems.

Health Problems

Health problems are categorized as acute, chronic, developmental, or cultural/environmental in nature. Acute and chronic health deviations are two major types of health problems. Problems of concern or interest to you may be chronic deviations such as congenital disorders, cardiovascular defects, rheumatoid arthritis, or drug dependency. You may respond well to the stress and changing status of critically ill clients in intensive care units (ICU). Acute deviations such as a myocardial infarction, infection, or accident may better suit you. You may want to focus on developmental problems such as the effects of smoking on pregnant women or sexual adjustments related to diabetes or spinal cord injury. You may value the importance of life events such as marriage, adolescence, empty nest, or retirement and focus on preventing health problems that these events may trigger.

You can explore practice options by reflecting on the type of health problem of interest to you. Consider how grave or important certain health problems are to you, keeping in mind personal characteristics, attributes, style, and stage. A nurse who relies on verbal interchange might eliminate a focus on developmental disabilities, aphasia, or other problems that limit verbal communication with patients. A nurse who values prevention might focus on nutrition problems of pregnant teens rather than respiratory problems of the person with chronic lung disease.

Human Response

Client responses to health problems consistently have been within the purview of nurses in practice and in theory building. Clients respond biologically, psychologically, and socially to health problems. Nurses intervene or support these response systems to promote effective, useful, and adaptive responses. Interventions address these response systems when clients are not functioning effectively on their own.

Nursing leaders and theorists share a common perspective in describing the kinds of client responses to which nurses attend. Henderson (1961) describes patient "functions" in physiologic and safety areas such as breathing, eating, and avoiding injury or social and psychologic areas such as play, work, and communication. Orem (1980) refers to six universal self-care "behaviors": intake, excretion, activity/rest, social interaction/solitude, safety, and normalcy. Roy (1976), identifies four distinct "modes," or ways, in which a person adapts or maintains integrity: the physiologic mode, the self-concept mode, the role function mode, and the interdependence mode. Loomis and Wood (1983) refer to six human response systems: physiologic, psychologic, cognitive, family, social, and cultural/environmental. For over a decade the National Conference on Clarification of Nursing Diagnosis has attempted to collect nursing diagnoses and organize them in a sensible and acceptable manner, using these and other theoretical schemes. Gordon (1982) organizes nursing diagnoses according to physiologic, psychologic, social, cognitive, and spiritual patterns. These are presented in Table 6–6.

You can focus practice on one or several of these response systems or patterns. Holism certainly necessitates considering all systems for any one client. However, you may have greater interest or skill in dealing with some systems than others. For instance, interest in what a person understands about a health problem focuses care on the client's cognitive response system; valuing social interaction focuses on the social support system. Nursing interventions are elicited when there is disequilibrium in any system and abnormal responses occur. The label placed on specific abnormal responses is a nursing diagnosis. Analyzing nursing diagnoses will help you describe a nursing focus.

TABLE 6–6   Grouping of Currently Accepted Diagnoses Under Functional Health Pattern Areas

1. Health-perception–health management pattern
   Noncompliance (specify)
   Injury, potential for
   Poisoning, potential for
   Suffocation, potential for
   Trauma, potential for

2. Nutritional–metabolic pattern
   Skin integrity, impairment of, actual
   Skin integrity, impairment of, potential
   Nutrition, alterations in, less than body requirements
   Nutrition, alterations in, more than body requirements
   Nutrition, alterations in, potential for more than body requirements
   Fluid volume deficit, actual
   Fluid volume deficit, potential

3. Elimination pattern
   Urinary elimination, alterations in patterns of
   Bowel elimination, alterations in: constipation
   Bowel elimination, alterations in: diarrhea
   Bowel elimination, alterations in: incontinence

4. Activity–exercise pattern
   Home maintenance management, impaired
   Self-care deficit (specify level): total
   Self-care deficit (specify level): feeding
   Self-care deficit (specify level): bathing/hygiene
   Self-care deficit (specify level): dressing/grooming
   Self-care deficit (specify level): toileting

   Airway clearance, ineffective
   Gas exchange, impaired
   Breathing pattern, ineffective
   Diversional activity, deficit in
   Tissue perfusion, alteration in (cerebral, cardiopulmonary, renal, gastrointestinal, peripheral)
   Cardiac output, alterations in: decreased

TABLE 6–6 *Continued*

---

5. Sleep–rest pattern
   Sleep pattern, disturbance in

6. Cognitive–perceptual pattern
   Knowledge deficit (specify)
   Sensory perceptual alterations (visual, auditory, kinesthetic, gustatory, tactile, olfactory)
   Comfort, alterations in: pain
   Thought processes, alterations in

7. Self-perception–self-concept pattern
   Fear (specify)
   Self-concept, disturbance in (body image, self-esteem, role performance, personal identity)

8. Role–relationship pattern
   Grieving, anticipatory
   Grieving, dysfunctional
   Parenting, alterations in: actual
   Parenting, alterations in: potential
   Communication, impaired verbal
   Violence, potential for

9. Sexuality–reproductive pattern
   Sexual dysfunction
   Rape–trauma syndrome
   Rape–trauma: compound reaction
   Rape–trauma: silent reaction

10. Coping–stress-tolerance pattern
    Coping, ineffective individual
    Coping, ineffective family: compromised
    Coping, ineffective family: disabling
    Coping, family: potential for growth

11. Value–belief pattern
    Spiritual distress (distress of human spirit)

Gordon M: *Nursing Diagnosis.* New York: McGraw-Hill, 1982.

The following exercise gives you an opportunity to describe the type(s) of health problems, response systems, and nursing diagnoses on which you want to focus your nursing practice.

Exercise 6–3 My Nursing Focus

1. Check the types of health problems that most interest you.

   _____ Acute health problems

   _____ Chronic health problems

   _____ Developmental life changes

   _____ Cultural or environmental stressors

2. List several specific health problems within the general category you checked that are of interest or concern to you.

   a. _____

   b. _____

   c. _____

   d. _____

3. Identify clients' response system(s) on which you really want to focus your practice. Ask yourself, "With what response system(s) am I most attuned?" Check what pertains and is highly preferred by you.

   _____ Physiologic

   _____ Psychologic/emotional

   _____ Cognitive

   _____ Social/family

   _____ Cultural

   _____ Spiritual

4. Refer to Table 6–6. Circle the nursing diagnoses, those specific abnormal responses to health problems, you most want to explore and work with in your career.

5. Check consistency between the diagnoses you circled and the response system(s) you checked in item 3. Describe your findings.

   _____

   _____

6. In a summary statement, describe your nursing focus:
   I really want to work with the health problem(s) of _____,

   focusing my energies on the clients's _____
   response system(s) and helping clients deal in particular with problems or nursing

   diagnoses such as _____

   _____

Nursing Function

You have probably noticed your individual strengths and weaknesses, preferences and dislikes for various types of nursing functions. To analyze fully and direct your nursing practice, it is useful to appreciate your attitudes and skill related to nursing function. Nursing function is analyzed by exploring four aspects: nursing process, treatment modality, proximity to client, and level of prevention. Each of these considerations assists you in your appreciation of yet another dimension of nursing options.

Nursing Process

Nursing process represents decision making applied to client care. Client needs are assessed and problems postulated for which a solution is tried. Although inherently dynamic and continuous, the process can be divided into five components: assessment, planning, implementation, evaluation, and documentation. Although all components are essential for effective problem solving, they need not be performed by one person. Naturally, some nurses are skilled and interested in all aspects of the process, but any one nurse may be more or less skilled in one particular component. Using the following descriptions, explore personal strengths and interests in each of these components.

Assessment and Diagnosis. Are you a "closet diagnostician?" Do you observe and abstract meaning from situations? Do you enjoy collecting data, doing nursing histories, interviewing clients' families, formulating tentative conclusions, and trying to support hunches with additional data from records and reports? (Refer to Exercises 5–2 and 5–7 in Chapter 5.) Do your perceived strength and preference for assessing and diagnosing correlate with your general theme? A strong interest in nursing assessment correlates with an investigative theme.

The nurse conducting health risk appraisals for a company offering employee health programs to large corporations should be skilled and interested in assessment. The nurse doing primary care as a nurse practitioner will consistently use physical examination and psychosocial assessment skills for effective sorting of clients for treatment or referral. The nurse researcher is the investigator par excellence.

Planning. Are you a person who takes the pieces of the puzzle, figures the overall picture, considers resources and time frames, and develops a plan for intervention and evaluation? Do you tend to formulate short- and long-term goals and objectives along with strategies that are workable and effective? Are you known for establishing priorities and making decisions about what is the best action to take? Do you often find yourself trying to clarify and pinpoint role expectations and responsibilities? (Again refer to Exercises 5–2 and 5–7.) A predominantly task-oriented and detailed style generally suits the persons involved in planning functions. Planning implies evaluation and research. The planner must establish criteria and methods to use in evaluating outcomes. Deciding the appropriateness of actions defined in the plan requires much investigation or use of research findings.

Both assessment and planning relate to the intellectual phase of nursing process. Orem (1980) distinguishes intellectual from technical and social methods of helping. Ask yourself if you are oriented to "thinking" kinds of work or practice and "doing" kinds of work.

Examples of nursing options that require much planning include the nurse in a government office of statewide planning and development, the nurse who is special projects director in a hospital, and the nurse doing instructional design. As nurses become more involved in developing new products and new delivery methods, more options for program planning certainly will evolve. Opportunities for planners will escalate both in single agencies and in multi-institutional systems.

Implementation.   Perhaps you favor providing the interventions, or carrying out the plan, and prefer to be less involved in front-end analysis or evaluation. Do you choose tasks such as managing patient care, making referrals, collaborating with health care professionals, teaching, changing dressings, monitoring? Are you the hands-on, action-oriented nurse? The strength of many nurses is this action orientation. Participating in the practical phase involves conducting and controlling therapeutic actions to address client or situation problems and needs.

The nurse with a focus on acute illness and physiologic processes often relies heavily on expedient and efficient implementation of both medical and nursing care plans. The nurse with expertise in implementing plans may be a clinician, teacher, or manager. A social or enterprising style typifies those who execute plans. However, a technologically oriented nurse, such as a nurse in charge of a uterine stress stimulation testing service, a nurse enterostomal therapist, or a dialysis nurse, would be inclined to a realistic style.

Evaluating.   Are you a strong critic, a "Monday-morning quarterback?" Do you spend much time analyzing and judging how well plans worked in addressing client or situation problems? Are you the one who poses questions such as "Are we reaching our goals?" or "Were we realistic with our plans?" or "Have we defined the problem well?" If so, you probably have skills and interest in the evaluation function.

An evaluator should be objective and have the ability to stand back and assess results of particular interventions. Evaluators make judgments on whether what is observed meets the criteria established. This role is especially difficult for nurses who are inclined to intervene, to show, to tell, and to instruct.

Nurses as teachers and supervisors are heavily involved in evaluating the care given by others. Often those in more indirect roles use and draw on evaluation skills. This function is exceedingly important in our era of budget justification, job retention, and program delineation. Indeed the future of many quality nursing products depends on the strength of evaluation skills of nurse designers. Nurses in quality assurance also rely on preference and skills in evaluating nursing care.

Documenting. Documentation is integral to the nursing process. Nursing assessment data and nursing notes document interventions and clients' progress toward problem resolution. The importance of well-written documentation becomes evident as records substantiate the need for care and appropriateness of reimbursement.

The writing function is a burden for some at the end of a clinical day, when the nurse faces many charts and resents the time involved. Some nurses value the written word and are able to organize ideas and write clearly. Some have skill better suited to fiction, writing poignantly and creatively to convey vivid images that evoke emotion. What often thwarts nurses' interest in writing is fear of peer ridicule and lack of confidence in the worth of ideas (Hall, 1983).

Just as documentation is receiving greater emphasis in clinical practice, writing nonfiction and fiction are gaining recognition as important and effective means of increasing professional power and positively influencing the image of nursing (Kalisch & Kalisch, 1984). Nurses' publications of practice suggestions, tips on health care, and opinions about the health care system advance client care, raise consumer awareness, and lead to needed reform. In fiction nurse-authors contribute to the changing image of the nurse from stereotypic handmaiden to autonomous, motivated, intelligent, and service-oriented professional. Writing opportunities for both fiction and nonfiction are numerous; nurses who seek power and influence and who express themselves well in writing might include this function in their nursing options.

Treatment Modality

Another method for analyzing nursing function is considering treatment modality. Appraising specific treatments that you perform well, enjoy, or prefer provides additional detail, so you can vary this dimension as you design nursing options.

Exercise 6—4   Level of Preference and Proficiency for Sample Treatments

Sample treatment skills, divided into types A, B, and C, are listed in the following boxes. For each skill, indicate your level of preference (1, low; 2, moderate; 3, high). Then appraise your current level of proficiency (1, advanced beginner; 2, competent; 3, proficient; 4, expert). Add your scores for both preference and proficiency, and write your totals in the spaces provided.

Type A Treatments	Preference			Proficiency			
Therapeutic touch	1	2	3	1	2	3	4
Skin care	1	2	3	1	2	3	4
Massage	1	2	3	1	2	3	4
Exercise	1	2	3	1	2	3	4
Providing comfort measures	1	2	3	1	2	3	4

Total: _____ + Total: _____ = _____
Score

Type B Treatments	Preference			Proficiency			
Biofeedback	1	2	3	1	2	3	4
One-to-one counseling	1	2	3	1	2	3	4
Cognitive restructuring	1	2	3	1	2	3	4
Lifestyle changes	1	2	3	1	2	3	4
Instructional classes	1	2	3	1	2	3	4

Total: _____ + Total: _____ = _____
Score

Type C Treatments	Preference			Proficiency			
Monitoring of vital signs and other parameters	1	2	3	1	2	3	4
Use of infection control	1	2	3	1	2	3	4
Legislating for health protection	1	2	3	1	2	3	4
Enterostomal therapy	1	2	3	1	2	3	4

Total: _____ + Total: _____ = _____
Score

Check the type of treatment skills with the highest scores.

_____Type A   _____ Type B   _____ Type C

There are subtle differences in the three groupings of treatment modalities in Exercise 6–4. Type A treatments infuse a client with new energies, resources, or things. These treatments are perceived as actions that are taken for the purpose of comforting and bolstering the client's own resources. Type B treatments are oriented to the client's development of new perceptions and methods for coping or adapting to the environment. Type C treatments are directed at modifying the environment. Bevis (1982) refers to these three types of nursing treatments as nurturative, generative, and protective. Lydia Hall differentiates care, or nurturing, interventions from core and from cure modalities (Hale & George, 1980). Nurturing treatments include hygienic and basic activities of daily living supports. Core treatments involve interpersonal use of self. Cure treatments entail implementation of medical orders. Orem (1980) differentiates three types of nursing systems similar to types of treatment modality: nursing actions in the wholly compensatory system, in the partially compensatory system, and in the supportive-education system. The guiding, supporting, and teaching interventions of Orem's supportive system are similar to Bevis' generative treatments, and Lydia Hall's core modalities.

Benner (1984) describes seven domains of nursing practice, including the helping role, teaching–coaching function, diagnostic and patient monitoring functions, managing rapidly changing situations, administering and monitoring therapeutic intervention and regimens, and functions related to quality and organizational and work roles. While describing the depth and complexity of nursing in interventions within these domains, Benner's overall categories, developed from a synthesis of nurses' accounts of their practice, demonstrate the differences between various modalities and the clusters of nursing treatment behaviors. Nursing includes many types of skills and treatments, providing a broad spectrum for choosing nursing interventions. It is up to you to assess preference and proficiency and to direct your career options toward utilizing the most suitable skills and treatments.

Proximity to Patient.   Another way to explore nursing function is to consider the proximity of nurse to client. Archer and Fleshman (1979) refer to three types of nursing services: direct, semidirect, and indirect.

Direct services require interaction or health care exchange with your client or client group. Do you prefer counseling or teaching, doing physical examinations, giving emergency care, and providing direct interventions to your clients? Semidirect services are care provided through others. A supervisor or teacher gives care through staff or students to clients. Some nurses prefer semidirect care because they enjoy guiding others' development of skills or knowledge. Indirect involvement is typified by the administrator, staffing coordinator, lobbyist, or health planner. Nurses in indirect roles are concerned with creating the systems within which other workers can function and optimally provide direct and semidirect care.

All three levels of proximity to clients are viable options. It is important for you to consider how close or how distant you want or need to be to the person actually receiving care.

Level of Prevention. Nurses usually are involved in some level of prevention. That level may be primary, secondary, or tertiary. Each level of prevention involves different emphases and functions. Primary prevention refers to health promotion and prevention of health problems or disease. Exercise classes, stress management, prenatal classes, and blood pressure screening are examples of primary preventive actions. Nursing actions directed toward prompt attention after disease or health problems are experienced are at a secondary level of prevention. The problems or health risks are apparent, and prevention is directed toward minimizing complications. Nurses in acute care settings more often attend to secondary levels of prevention. The third level of prevention includes rehabilitative nursing measures aimed at preventing further complications of chronic illnesses, accidents, or irreversible injuries. Helping clients develop new ways to manage their lives as a result of the residual effects of an illness or accident is the essence of tertiary prevention.

In assessing nursing function, consider the level of prevention that captures your interest. Reflect on your values and philosophy of health care. You may lean toward health promotion rather than disease prevention. On the other hand, because of life experiences and values, you may want to function in a role that emphasizes preventing further limitations or complications once disease has been experienced. Consider personal attributes such as knowledge and experience. Primary prevention requires understanding epidemiology, healthful lifestyles, and health teaching. Ask yourself what your needs and interests are in proximity to clients and treatment modalities. This gives clues to which type of prevention might be more suited to you. Level of prevention is one other way to describe nursing function and give dimension to your nursing practice options.

Exercise 6–5   Summary of Exploration of Nursing Functions

Circle the word(s) most appropriate to complete this summary of your exploration of nursing functions.

I would rather <u>assess/diagnose   plan   implement   evaluate   document</u> and focus my energies on treatment modalities that are
<u>nuturing   guiding   protective</u>, with proximity to patients that is
<u>direct   semidirect   indirect</u>, and an emphasis at a level of prevention that is
<u>primary   secondary   tertiary</u>.

Nursing functions are multiple and varied. You have seen the complex view you can take of this *one* dimension of nursing. Restructuring or designing your nursing option(s), considering this one dimension, will yield great personal and professional rewards.

Nursing Roles

The word role brings to mind a stage, a script, and an actor interacting with other players. *Role* in the context of nursing implies these elements: a sender, a place, expectations, and a receiver. A work role refers to a position and status with specific expectations or a job description for that position within an occupational sphere or a particular institution.

Pathways to practice have been designed in a comprehensive way by the Southern Regional Education Board in their nursing curriculum project (1982). Categories of nursing practice are presented in Figure 6–2. Review this grid carefully, noting the recommendations for education, the competencies, and roles that emerge as a nurse moves up clinical, research, administrative, or educative tracks.

Although general guidelines for particular nursing roles can be helpful, keep in mind that nursing roles are very fluid and are often unique to the settings in which they are enacted and to the individuals who enact them. Each institution or social system has its own goals, needs for service, rules, and regulations that influence the positions and expectations.

Roles are not only unique because of the way they are interpreted within a particular setting; they are also unique because of the role participants. Persons taking roles bring their own sets of behaviors, which are their personal expression and interpretation of job expectations. Based on personality, socialization in a role, and resources such as education, skills, and experience, each person shapes, adapts, or changes a role so that it is a unique way of interacting with others.

For career planning, it is necessary to assess the compatibility of role expectations with personal needs. For instance, the nurse who values altruism in the direct service of others may suffer role stress if expected to do budgets, coordinate programs, and keep records. Similarly, the nurse who wants to teach may resent having to do research, publish, and work on numerous committees.

The capabilities needed for a particular role must be consistent with personal resources. When capabilities in time or talent are exceeded, a person eventually suffers incompetence in a role. Conversely, when capabilities are not used and a nurse is overqualified for a role, discontent and unfulfilled potential results. Role success requires that you, your expectations for the role, your talents, and the skills required by the role are congruent.

Just as you should assess roles for setting, your personal expectations, and

Figure 6–2 Categories of nursing practice.

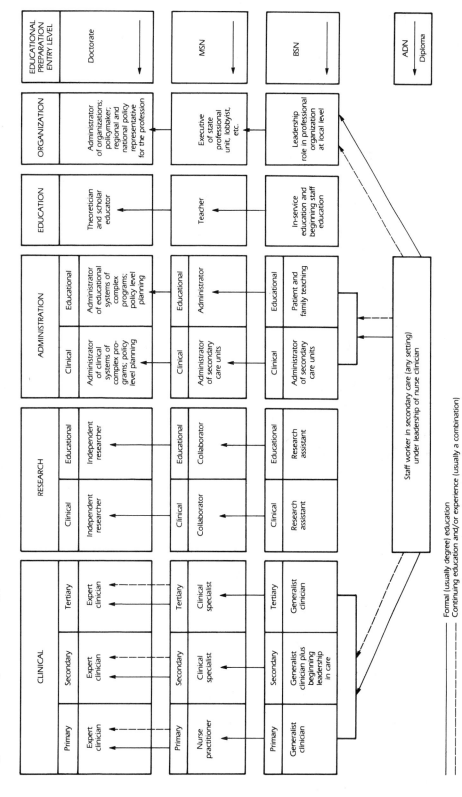

Reprinted from Southern Regional Education Board: *RN Education: The Basic Issues,* with permission.

——— Formal (usually degree) education
--------- Continuing education and/or experience (usually a combination)

your talents, you must maintain an awareness of their dynamic and constantly changing natures. You may assume a role that quickly evolves into a different role than you anticipated. Factors influencing role changes include changes in the organization, technology, societal roles, the economy, and legislation (Bullough, 1976; Christman, 1980).

An organization that changes from a nonprofit to a large corporate model with a for-profit component alters its overall goals and its expectations for many management and clinical roles. The nurse who had been delivering clinical care to clients in an ambulatory care setting may now be expected to develop for-profit educational programs and be faced with tremendous role change and possible dilemmas.

Technology can also create role impact. Nurses on medical units may be introduced to new medication administration equipment and be forced to alter interaction with the pharmacy and engineering departments. Nurses may have to use computers for client information storage and retrieval and to interact with other departments. These role changes influence the nature and timing of interaction with clients and other professionals as well as the extent of role satisfaction.

Gradual social changes affect nurses' expectations of the nature of the world. Nurses in leadership positions, desiring more power and prestige, may change the nature of nurse–physician interaction, the nurse–administrative role, and the nurse–client relationship. From a subordinate role, the career nurse can become a health care collaborator or colleague, a leader, and a powerful force in the system.

Economics have a great influence on roles. For instance, the prospective payment system for hospital reimbursement of Medicare can broaden the role expectations of the clinical nurse, requiring more ancillary functions or changing from a direct caregiver to an indirect supervisor of nonprofessional providers.

How any one state defines nursing practice in its Nurse Practice Act has a fundamental impact on the nursing role in that state. More nurses will seek role expansion as laws are refined within the states, and nursing diagnosis and treatment are provided for through expanded basic definition, regulatory law, standardized procedures, or through changes in the power of the physician to delegate these functions to the nurse.

A nursing role dynamically blends you, the system in which you work, and others with whom you interact in that system. Roles constantly evolve in response to organizational, societal, and legislative changes. Although you can glean general characteristics about nursing roles by considering the type of institution and common job expectations, comparing any two nurses in similar roles reveals great dissimilarities. Thumbnail sketches of various clinical, educational, administrative, research, and consultation roles are presented here, so that you can differentiate and further explore the many possibilities within this nursing dimension.

Clinical Roles

Clinical roles involve directly observing and treating clients. Approximately 80% of the 1.3 million employed registered nurses are involved in general nursing care (IOM, 1983) in hospitals or nursing homes. With the aging population and reimbursement limits for hospital care, opportunities will increase for clinical roles in community and home nursing.

Staff Nurse.   According to Haase (1976), the entry level staff nurse in a secondary care facility generally gives care to clients who are experiencing acute or chronic illness. The entry level staff nurse makes nursing judgments based on scientific knowledge but relies on procedures and standardized care plans. Interventions are directed toward alleviating biophysical and psychosocial health problems, the outcomes of which are usually predictable. As the staff nurse advances to level II, usually within 6 months to 1 year of practice, she or he relies less on standards and procedures and develops individual and innovative plans of care to meet specific client needs. A level II staff nurse with a broader base of experience cares for clients with complex and unpredictable problems.

Hospitals increasingly use clinical ladders to recognize and promote advancing nurses. A survey of clinical ladders (Huey, 1982) found that most have three to five steps that are differentiated by depth, scope, and/or increasing competencies usually related to use of nursing process, staff, and client education, leadership, and research. A model proposed by West (1983) integrates the clinical ladder with the management ladder. In this way clinical nurses at various levels have appropriate assignments and are accountable to a higher level clinician rather than a manager. Table 6–7 describes this four-level clinical ladder. The clinical nurse IV is the master clinician to whom the clinical

TABLE 6–7   Description/Levels of Nursing Practice

Level	Clinician
I	Beginning practitioner assigned to nursing unit
II	Practitioner with 1 to 3 years experience as staff nurse working in intensive nursing area or with acutely ill patient assignment, but still in staff position
III	Clinician with advanced assessment, planning, evaluation, and technical skills assigned to collaborate with one or more physicians and patient managers to coordinate care planning for a client case load
IV	Master clinician with advanced clinical planning skills assigned to coordinate clinical practice, recommend standards of practice and nursing policy. Research and development of new systems, quality control monitoring of clinical practice

Reprinted with permission from West ME: Keeping talented RNs in hospital practice. *Nurs Management* 1983; 14(8):38–44.

nurse III reports. In this system the clinical nurse III assumes responsibility for a caseload of roughly 25 clients, following them from a physician's office contact, through admitting, bed assignment, and care planning to writing nursing orders, evaluating effectiveness of the plan, and coordinating client discharge. The level II staff nurse implements the nursing plan of the clinical nurse III. This approach potentially increases revenues and markets both nursing services and the hospital because of the nurse–physician collaboration and continuity of nurse–client relationship.

In considering the rungs on clinical ladders, be aware of salary differentials. Salaries from the bottom to top rung of the clinical ladder typically differ by 43% but can differ by as much as 100% (Huey, 1982). Assess your needs for lateral movement also. Some ladders build administrative steps on the second or third clinical levels; others have no comparable administrative component or movement capability. As ladders become more refined and commonplace, rely on your career values, interests, and needs to guide your selection and progression.

Staff certification provides staff nurses with recognition of experience. Certification is available in many areas of practice: critical care, emergency care, nephrology, obstetrics, operating room, neurosurgical, psychiatric–mental health, medical–surgical, child–adolescent, neonatal intensive care, and nursing administration. Organizations granting the most certifications are the American Association of Critical Care Nurses (AACCN), the American Association of Nurse Anesthetists, and the American Nurses' Association. The 13 specialty organizations that grant certification and requirements are listed in the Appendix at the end of this chapter. The requirements for certification vary. Usual requirements for taking a certifying examination are a combination of 2 or more years' experience and completion of continuing education or specialized training. Misconceptions about specialty certification for specialty practice abound. A survey conducted by *RN* magazine (Lewis, 1984) indicated that many nurses refer to themselves as specialists if they have worked in an area other than medical–surgical units. In this survey only 13% were certified, a quarter of these by the AACCN. The rewards for certification in a specialty area include personal satisfaction, recognition by peers, and increased salary. Nurses choose certification based on needs and interests. With trends toward professionalism and accountability for the quality of care to consumers, certification undoubtedly will become more popular.

For the nurse who values direct client care, clinical nursing is one way to keep talents at the bedside and achieve clinical expertise. As acuity of clients increases, clinical nursing roles, especially in hospitals, will attract and require nurses with strengths in coordinating, technical skills, communicating, monitoring, and coping quickly with fluctuating conditions. Nurses who are able to advance on the clinical ladder or achieve certification will find many ways to grow in clinical roles.

Clinical Nurse Specialist. The clinical nurse specialist (CNS) has advanced expertise in a defined area of nursing, a specific focus, and a broad range of theories to apply to that area of practice. The current foci of the advanced clinical nurse are medical, surgical, and intensive care followed by concentrations in maternal–child health and psychiatric–mental health. The CNS is often at the top rung of clinical ladder structures. According to the document, *Nursing, A Social Policy Statement* (ANA, 1980), a clinical specialist is expected to

> observe, conceptualize, diagnose, and analyze complex clinical or nonclinical problems related to health, . . . consider a wide range of theory relevant to understanding those problems, and . . . select and justify application of theory deemed to be most useful in understanding problems and in determining the range of possible treatment options.

The clinical specialist practices with more autonomy, freedom, and self-discipline because of this high degree of expertise.

Clinical nurse specialists typically have responsibility in four areas: service, consultation, education, and research. Service involves identifying populations or communities at risk and providing sophisticated direct nursing care, often carrying a case load. Clinical specialists work with peers and other health care professionals, consulting on the planning and coordination of client care; they are expected to teach staff and clients formally and informally and participate to some degree in basic, graduate or continuing education; and they conduct research and translate findings into clinical practice. The research and investigative function also implies publishing findings. The future of clinical nurse specialists may lie in product line management, which includes clear product delineation, marketing, contract negotiation, and an emphasis on collaborating with physicians. Clinical nurse specialists are often hospital-based, but increasing numbers are found in public or community health, and home care.

The ANA criteria for clinical nurse specialists include an earned graduate degree and eligibility requirements for certification through the professional society. The title and role of the clinical nurse specialist can be confusing, however. Despite the ANA expectations for graduate preparation, only about 27% of 19,000 registered nurses holding the title in 1980 had attained graduate degrees; the rest are presumed to have completed some clinical specialty training offered through hospitals or continuing education departments of schools (IOM, 1983).

The Nurse Practitioner. The nurse practitioner (NP) emerged in the 1960s as a clinical entity, mainly to meet primary health care needs in underserved rural areas. In 1965 the first nurse practitioner program in pediatrics started in Colorado. In the 1970s thousands of nurses were trained by physicians for what, initially, were assistive medical roles. Preparation occurred through health agencies or medical and nursing school programs rather than through graduate nursing programs. Of the approximately 17,000 nurse practitioners and nurse midwives in 1980, 19% were prepared at the master's level (IOM, 1983). The number of practitioners with master degrees will increase as more graduate programs are offered.

Nurse practitioners, prepared beyond the basic level to assume expanded roles, predominantly conduct comprehensive assessments, make diagnoses, and are responsible for managing care of patients with common and well-defined health care problems, disabilities, or chronic illnesses. They conduct physical exams, often interpret laboratory tests and x-rays, and may perform special examinations such as vaginal exams to develop a broad data base. The nurse practitioner makes judgments about the health–illness status of clients, provides care and health counseling, and collaborates with other providers.

Some nurse practitioners have independent practices, providing care during regular office hours or making home visits. Most are employed in ambulatory care, with approximately 5600 in hospitals, 4500 in public or community health agencies and 4000 in physicians' offices or HMOs (IOM, 1983). In school settings nurse practitioners influence health behaviors in children and families through health education. In industry they introduce health maintenance programs and monitor hazards or stressors in the workplace. Nurse practitioners continue to attend to underserved populations. Approximately 23% work in inner cities and 22% work in rural areas (IOM, 1983). They more often practice and are certified in family care, pediatrics, maternal and child health, and adult and school nursing. In the future emphasis will be placed increasingly on the geriatric nurse practitioner providing long-term care in institutions and primary care in the home. Two major influences on their practice will be their success in procuring and maintaining third-party reimbursement and the supply of physicians by federal and state programs, especially those interested in family, geriatric, and primary care.

The role of nurse practitioners is not without strain. For example, while the nurse recognizes opportunity for a collegial and autonomous role, physicians often interpret the role as subordinate and ancillary. The blending of medical and nursing roles, with their differing but complementary perspectives, provides optimum team relationships and client care outcomes. This requires much negotiation and education. The legal boundaries established by state nurse and medical practice legislative acts dictate the degree of supervision or autonomy allowed the nurse practitioner. Employment of nurses for economic advantage implies that the practitioner role is a medical substitute rather than a distinct nursing service. Many of the nurse practitioner's traditional assessment and care management skills are integrated into other roles, such as clinical nurse specialist, which can confuse and obscure roles on the health care team.

Educational Roles

Educational roles include instructor or faculty in schools of nursing, staff development educator, or client educator in health agencies. Slightly more than 37,000 nurses are instructors in nursing education programs for generic or graduate degrees. An additional 16,000 nurses are in educational roles in hospitals and 2000 in nursing homes (IOM, 1983).

Faculty.   Educators in schools of nursing are responsible for lesson planning, instructing, and evaluating student learning. Faculty also advise assigned students on their programs of study and assist students in solving learning problems.

Most nursing schools require that faculty have advanced preparation. To teach baccalaureate or associate degree students, a master's degree in nursing is needed. As of June 1982, 19 states require a master's degree in nursing as the minimal preparation for senior faculty in all programs. Of the approximately 20,000 full-time nursing faculty members in 1980, only 7% have a doctorate degree and 68% have a master degree (IOM, 1983). To teach in a master's or doctoral program and some baccalaureate programs, a nurse needs a doctorate.

Many opportunities exist for faculty. Options are in content areas and levels of students, such as generic, experienced registered nurse, or graduate levels. Programs may be traditional or nontraditional, external or accelerated.

Roles and expectations of instructors vary tremendously, depending on the program level. At the vocational and associate level, weekly faculty meetings, committee meetings, some annual curriculum review, and work on reports for state and national accreditation are expected parts of the job. The teacher's major responsibility, however, is daily instruction in the classroom and/or on the clinical unit.

At the baccalaureate, graduate, or doctorate levels, faculty are faced with additional requirements for promotion and tenure. A faculty member generally moves from assistant, to associate, and then to full professor level.

Tenure describes a level or category where one's position is guaranteed until retirement. Intended to protect academic freedom, tenure does provide security and a sense of stability to faculty members who attain it. A faculty person has between 6 to 8 years to meet tenure requirements. Tenure and promotion requirements usually are a combination of teaching, expertise in clinical practice, community service, and scholarly activity. In a survey of 282 National League for Nursing–accredited baccalaureate programs, scholarly activity, especially in doctoral study, was rated more important in faculty member evaluation and for tenure (Baird et al, 1985).

No consensus has been reached on what constitutes scholarly activity. Smaller, private undergraduate programs place a higher value on public visibility activities such as awards, holding office in professional organizations, and speeches; institutions with graduate programs, health science centers, and larger universities rate publications (books, funded grant proposals, or research articles) as more important for promotion and attaining tenure.

Faculty positions are generally suited to persons who like to teach and study, who have a sense of commitment to the next generation of professionals, and who value formal academic preparation for practice. For some, a faculty position is practical, leaving summers free to pursue other interests, part-time clinical work, or research and providing needed breaks in routine. Especially at a college or university, salary is usually less than that at a health care agency for comparable experience.

Persons planning a faculty role should address problems related to earning a doctorate, struggling with promotion and tenure demands, and balancing teacher expectations with those for clinician, researcher, advisor, and community or professional member. The faculty role has much potential strain related to multiple relationships and expectations. Stressors include meeting concurrent student and client needs, evaluating and supervising students fairly, negotiating different theoretical viewpoints with other faculty members, presenting class content innovatively, researching, and meeting deadlines (Hinds et al., 1985). The faculty person gradually learns to blend and internalize the academic or professional educator role with the professional nurse role.

Staff Development. Nurses in staff development or in-service roles are responsible for the continued competence and advancement of nurses employed in a particular setting. The staff development educator has a dual focus: promoting opportunities for the growth of individual staff and supporting hospital and nursing service objectives and performance expectations. Depending on the health care agency and individual educator's philosophy, emphasis is placed on education for development, competency, or productivity. Staff development programs usually include continuing education, skills review, management development, and required in-services on products or procedures.

In addition to developing and teaching educational programs, staff development educators often assume a consultative function, facilitating department or group problem solving and planning. The nurse in staff development must form effective internal liaisons with key committees and external networks to keep apprised of needs, trends, advances, and resources available for programs or agency problem solving. Finally, the staff developer is responsible for efficiency and effectiveness of educational programs and services such as orientation, purchasing and cataloging of resources, educational needs assessment, and overall annual program planning.

Approaches for teaching in staff development are different from those used in academic settings. The learners are not a captive audience; the scheduling of classes is not at the teacher's or the department's convenience. Knowledge of adult learning theory is important for full appreciation of the performance problems and needs of the learners. A challenge to the staff developer is selecting and using effective, stimulating teaching approaches to hold the interest of busy employees and build on work and life experiences. Staff developers need consulting, coordinating, program planning, and budgeting skills.

The nurse educator in an acute care setting is prepared increasingly at the graduate level. For an assistant or clinical instructor role or teaching in the evening or on night shift, a baccalaureate degree may suffice. A basic value is education; interest in organizations and the people who work in them is a major characteristic required by a staff developer.

Health Educator.   The nurse who educates the consumer might work in a hospital or clinic, fitness center, weight reduction clinic, for a corporation, a group of physicians, or a television or cable company. The possibilities are limitless. The role requires strong teaching skills, interpersonal skills, persistence, and a willingness to be flexible in meeting consumer health education needs. A health educator should be able to communicate well, motivate the consumer, and place a high value on the consumer's participation in health care. A theory base in education and health promotion or disease prevention is needed to guide the content and approaches that are used.

Administrative Roles

Administrative roles in nursing service are those of first-line managers such as head nurses and executive managers such as directors. In many hospitals head nurses are responsible for single nursing care units, but supervisors are responsible for the overall management of several units. In some agencies the role of supervisor has been eliminated, with the head nurse answering directly to the director of nursing services.

Head Nurse.   Head nurses direct and develop nursing staff assigned to their units. They must control labor resources, establish budgets, and operate a given unit or service. Head nurses collaborate effectively with other departments and units within an agency. In addition, they supervise the implementation of standards, policies and procedures for quality client care. An effective nurse manager promotes a strong unit culture that coalesces with the department and the agency.

Director.   Depending on the size and complexity of the health care agency, the director of nursing services may be an assistant vice-president or even a vice-president. The director may be responsible to the vice-president or report directly to the chief executive officer. Directors of nursing services have overall control and responsibility for the nurses and nursing activities in their agency. Nurses in executive level positions establish department goals and objectives, plan programs, and administer budgets to meet the agency's goals. Senior level managers set policy and develop structures for operating units. Directors assume a broad organizational perspective and are the voice of their organization internally and in the community (Scott, 1984).

Nurses assume top administrative roles in hospitals, nursing homes, public or community health nursing settings, and schools of nursing. There are approximately 23,000 nurses in top administrative positions in hospitals and 20,000 in nursing homes. At the middle-management and supervisory level, nurses number approximately 49,000 in hospitals and 14,000 in nursing homes. Combined administrative and supervisory positions have 15,000 nurses in public and community health settings. There are 5000 deans and directors of nursing education programs (IOM, 1983).

The education of nurses in top administration is generally at the baccalaureate level or above. In agencies of 300 beds or less nursing administrators are more often prepared at the baccalaureate level. Approximately 18% of top administrators are prepared at the master's level, with 1.4% prepared at the doctoral level (IOM, 1983). Interestingly, a study of Magnet Hospitals revealed that in those hospitals reported as positive places for nurses to work, nearly 70% of directors had master degrees and more than 12% had doctorates. (Schull, 1984).

Nurses considering administrative positions need a strong knowledge base in management practices, including theory related to change, decision making, finance, marketing, and personnel management. Theory and knowledge depend on skill, strengths, and experiences. Nurses in administrative roles must be skilled in fact-finding, analyzing, advice seeking, listening, and negotiating (Conway, 1974). In the current social environment a manager must be able to adapt to consumer demands, economic restraint, political environment, and technologic changes. For example, the administrator in an educational institution must guide and support faculty in developing programs that serve increasingly older students, incorporate more computer, video-supported, and home courses, search for private funding, and gain membership and influence on health and education committees at all levels of government.

Nurse managers are expected to exhibit qualities of risk taking, assertiveness, self-reliance, and achievement orientation. Traditionally viewed as masculine, success related to these qualities, is reported as more prevalent among women with mentors, those with strong paternal ties, and with coeducational school experiences (Krueger, 1980). The human-relations, coaching, and compassionate approaches, which women in management offer, combine with these so-called masculine qualities to present a new, perhaps optimum, management style.

Management ladders delineated in many agencies provide graded experiences from charge nurse to head nurse and from assistant to full director. Table 6–8 describes these levels of practice (West, 1983). In addition to following formal programs and ladders to become an administrator, a nurse gains invaluable skills through special assignments or project work, involvement in unit budgets, and informal networking with the management team.

Nurse managers require knowledge, preparation, and appropriate experiences and characteristics. Once these requirements are met, nurse management

TABLE 6–8   Description/Levels of Nursing Practice

Level	Administrative
I	Beginning practitioner assigned to nursing unit
II	Practitioner with 1 to 3 years experience as staff nurse working as charge nurse or relief charge nurse more than 20 hours per week
III	Practitioner with leadership management skills maintaining 24-hour accountability for patient care delivery for specific cost center. Includes total responsibility for all patient management activities and supervision of all permanently assigned personnel
IV	"Manager of Managers" with executive level ability to plan, organize and control assigned cost centers; knowledge of managerial theory/practice, labor resource management, budgeting and other managerial skills

Reprinted with permission from West ME: Keeping talented RNs in hospital practice. *Nurs Management* 1983; 14(8):38–44.

roles can offer power, recognition, prestige, and economic gain. A great amount of personal satisfaction stems from working with nurses as they reach quality client care standards and attain department or unit objectives. The scope of responsibility, pressures of competition, hard work, and high degree of flexibility are challenges for many.

Research Roles

The nurse researcher clarifies questions, systematically seeks answers within a larger theoretic framework, and presents them for the scrutiny of others. A researcher often is responsible for developing proposals for funding research projects as well as for actually conducting the research proposed.

The researcher's goal is to develop and test theories that will help explain and predict events and solve problems. A researcher may focus on natural, biologic, physical, or psychosocial sciences.

Some clinical ladders specify involvement in research as a criterion for advancement from staff nurse III to clinical nurse specialist. In other career ladders a separate research track allows progression from assistant to independent research roles. The person in an independent academic or service research role, however, is usually prepared at the doctoral level. Of the 3000 nurses employed in 1980 who had a doctorate degree, only about 6% were primarily engaged in research (IOM, 1983). Research roles require strong observation, communication, and statistical and analytical skills. Researchers work painstakingly, reviewing the literature, setting up observational or experimental opportunities, or probing for patterns in collected data, records, or documents. They must be systematic, detailed, persistent, inquisitive, tolerant of ambiguity, and open to the scrutiny of others.

Opportunities in nursing research, focusing on major issues such as the cost-effectiveness of alternate delivery systems, clinical and health care concerns, nursing interventions, and consumer coping behaviors, are timely and exciting. Meaningful rewards for nurse researchers include gaining the power of expertise and the opportunity for professional and social contributions.

Although traditionally hired by schools of nursing, researchers are being hired by large medical centers and medium-sized hospitals. Roles exist not only in traditional clinical research, but also in program evaluation, quality assurance, and administrative consultation, where research methodologies are applicable and increasingly valued. As more nursing research moneys become available and the perceived value of research is validated by productive and cost-related outcomes, nursing research roles will undoubtedly proliferate. More nurse researchers, prepared and skilled in competing for research grants, will be employed and become highly valued for the prestige, revenues, and insights that grants can provide their agencies, staff, and clients.

Consultation Roles

A consultant role is one of expert advisor. Consultants use special technical knowledge and skill in tasks such as computer systems development, skills training, or theory evaluation. A consultant may be a process expert, facilitating an organization's or group's problem-solving techniques. A process consultant offers fewer answers and raises more questions in an attempt to help the client strengthen internal capabilities. A hospital, attempting to develop esprit de corps within its nursing department, might contract with a nurse specialist to conduct a series on group dynamics, communication, conflict management, and negotiation. Another agency with a similar need for team building might contract for a process consultant to assess problems or barriers and recommend a plan of action.

Consultants often assume many separate roles such as clinical nurse, teacher, technologist, counselor, or even researcher to accomplish a task or solve a problem. A distinguishing characteristic of consulting is that it is a time-limited contract with an organization or group; it is a temporary interaction between the consultant and the system. The value of the consultant is often in the development of human potential. As an outside observer, the consultant can be effective in objectively assessing a situation and implementing cost-efficient solutions.

Consultants are usually prepared at the master's level or higher. If well prepared, they can draw on various theories related to group process, teaching–learning process, organizational theories, and role theory as well as specific knowledge and skill. An independent consultant needs marketing and networking skills to attract and win contracts. Some consultants, however, are employees of large firms that handle the bidding and community image aspects of the business.

When independently employed, a consultant must be flexible, creative, and confident. Benefits of consulting include prestige, independence, and varied work projects. Also, earning potentials are high with ranges of $30,000 to $50,000 annual salaries, often with stock options and appealing benefits packages if employed by industry or consulting firms (Wells, 1984). Disadvantages of consulting are instability of contracts, a feeling of "rootlessness," moving from agency to agency and job to job. Consultants can become trapped in nonproductive work by clients who use them to justify predetermined changes rather than to consider options.

Roles and Role Configurations

Many nursing roles have not been defined here, including nurse politician, nurse recruiter, quality assurance coordinator, infection control nurse, and budget or systems analyst. Some roles intersect with other fields such as medicine, business, law, and government. Nurses combine roles and assume new ones such as lobbyist, consumer advocate, or lawyer. At times individual nurses cross into apparently less related fields such as the arts to develop unique roles as nurse humorist, dance therapist, sign linguist, or image enhancer.

Influences on the expansion or creation of new nursing roles include legislation, methods of payment, consumer demands, consumer expectations, and individual expertise and ability to assume or create new roles. Roles for nursing are not fixed. Sharp role delineation into clinical, research, administration, education, or consultation areas is rare and probably inappropriate for most nurses and settings. For instance, in clinical roles, the nurse often researches and educates. The role of the clinical nurse specialist merges the roles of clinician, educator, and researcher. Increasingly, dual appointments between education and service settings are being established. In joint education–service appointments, a nurse is a faculty member and concurrently a clinical specialist in the service setting. The multifunctional approach to roles, as proposed by Baker (1981), is compared with traditional nursing functions in Figure 6–3. The professional academician combines all three roles of teacher, practitioner, and researcher. The professional practitioner, the mentor, and the traditional teacher each merge two of the three functional areas.

You may find that your nursing role will be an individual configuration of various functions in a particular system. For instance, you may function as a faculty person in an academic setting, act as a project director for an innovative educational outreach effort, and simultaneously be an independent consultant for nursing service in the area of instructional design. For you, a role label like "nursing education specialist" would unify these various functions in multiple settings. Regardless of whether your role is delineated, or combines multiple functions, it is important that you establish a clear perception of your preferences and interests in that role.

Figure 6–3 Nursing functions. TA, traditional academician (researcher, teacher); PA, professional academician (teacher, practice, researcher); PP, professional practitioner (practice, research); CM, clinical mentor (practice, teacher)

Current nursing functions

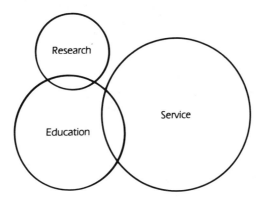

Optimum multifunction approach

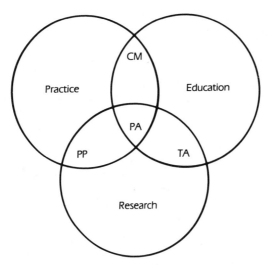

From Baker C: Interdependence: Strategies for collaboration. *J Nurs Admin* (April) 1981;11:34–39, with permission.

Exercise 6–8 Preferences for Typical Roles

1. Indicate your preferences for the following nursing roles (1, low; 2, moderate; 3, high).

Role	*Preference*		
a. Clinical	1	2	3
b. Educational	1	2	3
c. Administrative	1	2	3
d. Research	1	2	3
e. Consultation	1	2	3
f. Other	1	2	3

2. Describe or give an example of those you rated highest. For instance, if an educational role is preferred, is it consumer health educator, faculty member, or trainer? If you rated consultant and "other" as high preferences, write your unique combination such as consultant and therapist, biologist, or lawyer.

    a. Role(s) _____

    Description and examples:_____

    _____

    _____

    _____

    _____

    b. Role(s): _____

    Description and examples: _____

    _____

    _____

    _____

3. List the rewards and requirements for the role(s) you have described.
    Role a

    Rewards: _____

    Requirements: _____

    Role b

    Rewards: _____

    Requirements: _____

Comment on the consistency of your personal attributes and the characteristics, style, and stage with these roles.

_____

_____

_____

_____

A Synthesis: Professional Goals

Up to this point you have analyzed nursing very closely. You have investigated nursing role, functions, health problems and client responses, and various client and setting possibilities for your career. This is a first step on the road to designing your meaningful professional goals; the next step is synthesis. Synopses of several nurses' practices show how they synthesized these dimensions.

Exercise 6–9   Identifying Dimensions of Practice

Read the following case examples of nurses' practices. As you read, try to identify the six major dimensions of nursing practice. Check in the spaces provided (Yes or No) whether you believe the dimension has been described by the nurse.

Case Example: Nurse A

I am a nurse practitioner in the pediatric oncology department of a large teaching hospital. I work with a team of oncologists and surgeons.

The babies or children on our unit have Wilm's tumor, brain tumors, leukemias, and all types of cancer that affect children. I work mainly with familes, helping them understand the diagnosis and teaching them how to care for their child, including how to administer, monitor, and treat the side effects of their medications. I assess parents as they support the child's growth and offer them guidance in how to approach their child about the disease, its meaning, and treatments. When a child needs to go to the hospital for tests or surgery, I make home visits to prepare the family for this experience.

Dimensions	Described in this case?
Client	Yes _____ No _____
Site	Yes _____ No _____

Dimensions	Described in this case?	
Health problem	Yes _____	No _____
Human response	Yes _____	No _____
Nursing functions	Yes _____	No _____
Nursing role	Yes _____	No _____

Case Example: Nurse B

I work in the field of developmental disabilities. In that field I am a generalist among specialists, playing a pivotal role within an interdisciplinary team for children and families. I have established an independent practice and see clients in my office and make home, school, or other agency visits. I work with children with diagnoses such as mental retardation, cerebral palsy, epilepsy, and learning disabilities. My focus is helping parents learn how to cope with the unending nature of developmental limitations and with their own grief.

My practice grew out of the realization that someone was needed outside of any one system to really assist families in making the best use of their own resources in these kinds of situations. I focus my practice on increasing parent competence. I assist families in examining problems, discovering new options and strategies, mainly through parent counseling and use of behavior analysis and behavior modification techniques. In addition, I refer clients, assist them with using community resources, and often act in an advocacy position for them.

Dimensions	Described in this case?	
Client	Yes _____	No _____
Site	Yes _____	No _____
Health problem	Yes _____	No _____
Human response	Yes _____	No _____
Nursing functions	Yes _____	No _____
Nursing role	Yes _____	No _____

It is evident from Case Examples A and B that nursing practice takes varied forms. The dimensions that both nurses describe reflect and affect the whole of their nursing practices. Both nurses have clinical nursing roles, one as nurse practitioner, the other as independent practitioner. One works in a hospital setting, the other in a private office. The focus of their practices is on chronic health problems related to disease or developmental disabilities. The family as both client and response system is the major emphasis for both nurses. Nursing functions in both cases include counseling and teaching interventions. Review the next case, noting how different the nurse's role, functions, and focus are from the previous cases.

Case Example: Nurse C

I am a nurse supervisor and a family nurse practitioner for a county detention facility. I do direct client/inmate assessments, diagnosis, referral, and treatment of common medical and psychiatric illnesses; I share this responsibility with the medical supervisor for the facility. In addition, I supervise 14 nurses on staff in the care and treatment of inmates for three facilities. This involves scheduling and evaluating their professional performances, providing the opportunity for group conflict resolution, and offering continuing education programs. I define and monitor professional nursing standards of practice at the facilities and have been involved over the years in formulating and implementing all of the county policies and procedures in accordance with the national jail accreditation body. I meet with the department heads on a monthly basis from many county offices to represent the jail medical services. As a group, we are involved in problem solving, developing policies for various services, and dealing with county issues associated with disaster planning, food services, and material procurement.

As a nurse practitioner, I do enjoy the investigative aspects of health care such as differential diagnosis, but I also like research. For instance, I am now developing a grant proposal for comparing the health care problems of narcotic addicts in private care to those in government detention facilities. My job often has involved me in special projects such as a rubella-titer project and task analysis studies that helped justify my staffing recommendations for our jail system.

You can see that my job is extremely diversified, and I love it! I value this kind of variation and am involved in travel and study tours as well as archeologic digs during my summer vacation time.

Dimensions	Described in this case?	
Client	Yes _____	No _____
Site	Yes _____	No _____
Health problem	Yes _____	No _____
Human response	Yes _____	No _____
Nursing functions	Yes _____	No _____
Nursing role	Yes _____	No _____

Take the time to identify, describe, and rank your preferences in each of the six dimensions. You may want to refer to the notations you made in this chapter, or just jot down your thoughts now and later check consistency or elaborate on each dimension.

Exercise 6—9 Describing and Setting Your Nursing Dimension and Priorities

Based on your review and reflections in this chapter, list three of your perceptions, completing the statements for each nursing dimension provided here. Then rank your priorities within each dimension from most to least preferred (1, most preferred; 2, moderately preferred; 3, least preferred). Place the appropriate number in the space provided next to each option.

I see myself **focused** on these **health problems and human responses:**

	Dimension	*Priority*
a.	_____	_____
b.	_____	_____
c.	_____	_____

Doing these kinds of **functions:**

	Dimension	*Priority*
a.	_____	_____
b.	_____	_____
c.	_____	_____

For these **clients:**

	Dimension	*Priority*
a.	_____	_____
b.	_____	_____
c.	_____	_____

In these **settings:**

	Dimension	*Priority*
a.	_____	_____
b.	_____	_____
c.	_____	_____

And practicing in these **roles:**

	Dimension	*Priority*
a.	_____	_____
b.	_____	_____
c.	_____	_____

From your lists of priority options, you will synthesize your descriptions to obtain your professional goals. These goals will evolve by looking at your nursing practice from a broader perspective and from your investigation of the six dimensions of nursing and the array of nursing options available.

Exercise 6–10 Designing Professional Goals

Referring to the descriptions of the nursing dimensions from Exercise 6–9, combine priorities to determine individual nursing goals that reflect your preferences for various nursing dimensions. Describe at least three different nursing goals by combining the dimensions that you have written. Combine your high priority items, your moderate preferences, and your lowest priority items. Do not let tradition or concern of the practical impede your work here. Your options may be quite novel. Now is the time to be creative and free with your choices. Reality testing and assessing outcomes are the next stages of the process, and are considered in Chapters 7 and 8. For now, complete the phrase for each of your nursing goals.

Goal I: I see myself

_____

_____

_____

Goal II: I see myself

_____

_____

_____

Goal III: I see myself

_____

_____

_____

_____

The last steps of synthesis involve matching professional goals with personal goals. It is important to apply the elements from your self-examination to your nursing options. It is wise to assess the mesh of your personal characteristics, stage, style, and attributes with your preferred nursing options. The maximum match of self with professional directions results in career satisfaction and vitality.

One nurse, Stacy, listed the following personal characteristics: high value for expertise; believing in "an ounce of prevention," monetary rewards; an interest in the great outdoors and enjoyment of spectator sports; strong skills in working with data; secondary skills in persuading and selling, and preference for investigative style. He designed one professional goal as follows: "I want to work with elderly clients in a rural hospital, focusing on the emotional problems of the physically immobilized client, and primarily practicing one-to-one or small-group counseling as a psychiatric clinical specialist."

In comparing Stacy's personal characteristics with his preference for nursing options, a blend exists in some areas but not in others. The skills preference for working with data might be expanded so that research is done as well as counseling. With his preference for investigative style, a hospital setting needs to be assessed carefully for management style and support for nurses. Interest in the outdoors could be emphasized in other aspects of life, but the hospital setting dimension does not seem to fit Stacy that well. Values are also inconsistent. A strong health promotion philosophy might put him at odds with the tertiary level of care.

Lining up personal characteristics with nursing options forces you to analyze further the degree of consistency and integration of your nursing practice option with personal goals. It also encourages you to adapt or adjust either the nursing options or other aspects of work or life for maximum career and self-realization.

Exercise 6–11   Confirming That Professional Goals Match Personal Traits

In column A list three descriptions of your major personal traits that you assessed in Exercise 5–15 in Chapter 5. In column B give a thumbnail sketch of the three nursing goals that you have designed in Exercise 6–10. Look at both lists carefully.

Assess the blend of personal traits with your nursing goals. Use the blanks provided to indicate presence of a match (check Yes or No). Make some decisions about whether adaptations are needed in your nursing or personal goals.

Column A: traits   *Column B: goals*

A. Characteristics   GOAL I:

_____   _____

_____   _____

_____   Blend of traits A: Yes _____ No _____

B. Attributes

_____

_____

_____

C. Style

_____

_____

_____

D. Stage

_____

_____

_____

B: Yes _____ No _____

C: Yes _____ No _____

D: Yes _____ No _____

Adequate rewards: Yes _____ No _____

Meet requirements: Yes _____ No _____

<u>GOAL II:</u>

_____

_____

Blend of traits A: Yes _____ No _____

B: Yes _____ No _____

C: Yes _____ No _____

D: Yes _____ No _____

Adequate rewards: Yes _____ No _____

Meet requirements: Yes _____ No _____

<u>GOAL III:</u>

_____

_____

Blend of traits A: Yes _____ No _____

B: Yes _____ No _____

C: Yes _____ No _____

D: Yes _____ No _____

Adequate rewards: Yes _____ No _____

Meet requirements: Yes _____ No _____

Explore your findings, areas of consistency, and any apparent inconsistencies. What have you discovered? Comment on personal and professional adjustments you would make.

_____

_____

_____

Discuss this exercise with two other persons, preferably a significant other and a professional colleague.

Note any further inconsistencies and areas of strong validation from others.

_____

_____

_____

You have implemented a structure for analysis of nursing options. Using six key dimensions—client, setting, health problem, human response system, nursing role, and function—you have explored nursing and developed several goals. As you reviewed each dimension, you considered your personal considerations, options, stage, and style and applied this to your nursing analysis.

Congratulations on a process systematically and thoroughly done. What has evolved are statements of professional goals that have been checked against your personal profile. As you continue, you will be rewarded by the ensuing confidence that a full exploration of information about nursing has on your career planning. These professional goals are still tentative. With further reality testing against trends and common practice and with additional evaluating, your career goals will emerge as highly probable and realistic.

References

As controversy mounts over hospitals-for-profit. *USNWR* (Dec) 1984; 97:61–62.

Archer S, Fleshman R: *Community Health Nursing*, p. 461. North Scituate, MA: Duxbury Press, 1979

Baird S et al: Defining scholarly activity in nursing education. *J Nurs Educ* (April) 1985; 24:143–147.

Baker C: Moving toward interdependence: Strategies for collaboration. *J Nurs Admin* (April) 1981; 11:34–39.

Benner P: *From Novice to Expert*, pp. 39–46. Menlo Park, CA: Addison-Wesley, 1984.

Bevis E: *Curriculum Building in Nursing: A Process*, pp. 49; 141. St. Louis, MO: Mosby, 1982.

Bullough B: Influences on role expansion. *AJN* 1976; 76(9): 1476–1481.

Carr E: A model for private practice. In: *Socialization, Sexism and Stereotypes*, pp. 413–423. Muff J (editor) St. Louis: Mosby, 1982.

Christman L: Problems of role definition in the health care team. In: *Current Perspectives in Nursing*, pp. 15–23. Flynn B, Miller M (editors). St. Louis: Mosby, 1980.

Coleman J, Dayani E, Simms E: Nursing careers in the emerging systems. *Nurs Management* 1984; 15(1): 26.

Conway ME: Management effectiveness and the role-making process. *J Nurs Admin* 1974; 416:Nov/Dec, 25–28.

Deal T, Kennedy A, Spiegel A: How to create an outstanding hospital culture. *Hosp Forum* 1983;26(1):21–28; 33–34.

Fawcett J: A framework for analysis and evaluation of conceptual models of nursing. *Nurse Educ* 1980; 5:10–14.

Fawcett J: The paradigm of nursing: present status and future requirements. *Image 1984; 16(3):84–87.*

Gordon M: *Nursing Diagnosis,* pp. 327–328. New York: McGraw-Hill, 1982.

Haase P: Pathways to practice. *AJN* 1976; 76(6):950–954.

Hale K, George J: Lydia E. Hall. In: *Nursing theories: The base for professional nursing practice,* pp. 39–48. Englewood Cliffs, NJ: Prentice-Hall, 1980.

Hall S: Publishing as a source of power. In: *Power and Influence: A Source Book for Nurses,* pp. 151–185. Stevens K (editor). New York: Wiley, 1983.

Henderson V: *Basic Principles of Nursing Care.* London: International Council of nurses, 1961.

Hinds P et al: Self-identified stressors in the role of nursing faculty. *J Nurs Educ* 1985 (Feb); 24(2): 63–68.

Huey F: Looking at ladders. *AJN* 1982 (Oct); 82(10):1520–1526.

Ingalls J: *Human Energy, the Critical Factor for Individuals and Organizations,* pp. 50–53. Austin, TX: Learning Concepts, 1976.

Institute of Medicine: *Nursing and Nursing Education: Public Policy and Private Actions,* pp. 27; 44; 134; 136–137; 139; 215. Washington, DC: National Academy Press, 1983.

Kalisch B, Kalisch P: Improving the image of the nurse through nurse-authored novels. *Stanford Nurse* 1984; Fall:6–9.

Kinlein ML: *Independent Nursing Practice with Clients.* San Jose, CA: Lippincott, 1977.

Krueger J: Women in management: an assessment. *Nurs Outlook* 1980; 28:374–378.

Lewis HR: Specialism: the best career path? *RN* 1984; 47(6):40–47.

Loomis M, Wood D: Cure: the potential outcome of nursing care. *Image 1983; 15(1):4.*

Malanka P: Reaching for excellence: a look at what nursing can do. *Nurs Life* 1984; 4(3):41–46.

McClure M et al: Task force on nursing practice in hospitals of American Academy of Nursing. In: *Magnet Hospital Attraction and Retention of Professional Nurses.* Kansas City, MO: American Nurses' Association, 1983.

Muff J: Joint practice. In: *Socialization, Sexism and Stereotyping*, pp. 378–383. Muff J (editor). St. Louis: Mosby, 1982.

Nurses today: A statistical portrait. *AJN* 1982; 82:448–451.

Nursing: A Social Policy Statement, pp. 9; 29. Kansas City, MO: American Nurses' Association, 1980.

Orem D: *Nursing: Concepts of Practice*, pp. 35–51; 96–101; 104–109. New York: McGraw-Hill, 1980.

Ort S, Putt A: *Teaching in Collegiate Schools of Nursing*, pp. 227–229. Boston: Little Brown, 1985.

Roy C: *Introduction to Nursing: An Adaptation Model.* Englewood Cliffs, NJ: Prentice-Hall, 1976.

Schull P: Magnet hospitals: why they attract nurses. *Nurs 84* 1984; 14(10):50–51.

Scott P: Executive career planning. *Nurs Econ* 1984; 2:62.

Simms E: Preparation for independent practice. *Nurs Outlook* 1977; 25:114.

Southern Regional Education Board: *RN programs: the right of passage. 1.* Pathways to practice. RN Education: *The Basic Issues.*

Sovie M: Economics of magnetism. *Nurs Econ* 1984; 2:85–92.

Wells P: The nurse consultant. *Imprint* 1984; 31(4):23–24.

West ME: Keeping talented RNs in hospital practice. *Nurs Management* 1983; 14(8):38–44

Williamson J: Master's education: a need for nomenclature. *Image* 15 (4):99–101.

Wilson HS: *Research in Nursing*, pp. 13–15. Menlo Park, CA: Addison-Wesley, 1985.

You mean a nurse owns this company? *Calif Nurse,* 1984; 80:6–7.

Appendix

Certificates for Specialist Registered Nurses

This study has identified 13 certifying organizations reporting special certification for 69,140 registered nurses (RNs), of whom 13,593 are nurse practitioners and nurse midwives. The following tables list these organizations together with relevant information. Table 1 lists all identified nurse certifying organizations. Tables 2 and 3 contain information on two organizations that certify RNs in specialty areas. In all tables, certification for nurse practitioners/nurse midwives is underlined. The information was obtained from members of the National Federation for Specialty Nursing Organizations and American Nurses' Association publications in November 1982.

TABLE 1 All Identified Nurse Certifying Organizations

Organization	Year Began Certifying	Total Number Certified	Eligibility Requirements for Certification
American Nurses' Association (ANA)	1974	10,269[a]	(Detail in Table 2)
American Association of Critical Care Nurses (AACN)	1976	12,101	RN licensure 1 year of critical care experience within past 3 years
American Association of Nurse Anesthetists (AANA)	1946	~19,000	RN licensure Graduation from approved program in nurse anesthesia
American College of Nurse Midwives (ACNM)	1971	2598	RN licensure Graduation from approved program in nurse midwifery

[a]Does not include those jointly certified with NAACOG, but does include nurse practitioners.

Organization	Year Began Certifying	Total Number Certified	Eligibility Requirements for Certification
Association of Operating Room Nurses (AORN)	1979	3770	RN licensure 2400 hours of practical experience in operating room within the last 2 years Must be recertified every 5 years
Emergency Department Nurses Association	1980	6000	RN licensure 2 years of emergency room experience is recommended
Nurses' Association of the American College of Obstetrics and Gynecology (NAACOG)	1975	3968	(Detail in Table 3)
American Board of Neurosurgical Nurses	1977	1120	RN licensure 2 years of experience preferably in the field
American Association of Occupational Health Nurses (AAOHN)	1972[b]	2406	RN licensure 5 years of experience in occupational health nursing 60 contact hours of continuing education within last 5 years Currently employed full time in occupational health nursing
American Board of Urologic Allied Health Professionals	1972	~500; "a few" LPNs	RN or LPN or physician's assistant licensure Employed in urology for at least 1 year prior to examination
International Association for Accredited Enterostomal Therapy	1979	608	RN licensure Graduate of a 6- to 8-week enterostomal therapy course Practice as an RN for at least 2 years prior to attending enterostomal course
Board of Nephrology Field Examiners	1977	~4000	RN licensure Currently employed in 1 year of clinical experience in field
National Board of Pediatric Nurse Practitioners and Associates	1977	2800	RN licensure Graduation from a formal pediatric nurse practitioner program

[b]The AAOHN began certifying occupational health nurses in 1972. From 1972 until 1974, those nurses desiring certification were "grandfathered" in. The first occupational health nursing certifying exam was given in 1974.
Reprinted from Nursing and Nursing Education: Public Policies and Private Actions, with permission of the National Academy Press, Washington, DC, 1983.

TABLE 2 American Nurses' Association Specialty Certification

Title of Specialty Area	Total Number Certified	Eligibility Requirements for Certification
Adult clinical specialist (psychiatric and mental health nursing)	731	MSN in psychiatric and mental health nursing Currently employed in direct patient care at least 4 hours each week Post-MSN practice in field at least 8 hours per week for 2 years or 4 hours per week for 4 years Experience in at least 2 different treatment modalities 100 hours post-MSN supervision Access to clinical supervision or consultation
Child and adolescent specialist (psychiatric and mental health nursing)	66	As above
Psychiatric and mental health nursing	633	Currently practicing in field giving direct patient care at least 4 hours per week Have practiced 24 of the last 48 months in the field Have access to supervision or consultation
Medical-surgical nursing	437	Currently practicing in field giving direct patient care at least 16 hours per week Have practiced 24 of last 36 months in field an average of at least 16 hours per week
Medical-surgical clinical specialists	154	MSN Currently practicing in field giving direct patient care an average of at least 4 hours per week Have practiced 12 of last 24 months as clinical specialist (post MSN) giving direct patient care an average of at least 16 hours per week
Child and adolescent nursing	95	1500 hours of direct patient care in maternal and child health Provided at least 200 hours of direct nursing care to children and adolescents 2 of last 3 years 30 contact hours of continuing education in field within last 3 years
Gerontology nursing	492	2 years of practice as a gerontologic nurse
Nurse administration	1119	Currently in middle management or executive nursing administrative position Have been in middle or executive level nursing administrative position at least 24 months within last 5 years Documentation of administrative responsibilities
Nurse administration advanced	413	Master degree Currently in executive level nursing administration or providing consultation in same Have worked in executive level nursing position or provided such consultation at least 36 months within last 5 years Documentation of administrative responsibilities
Community health nursing	218	Have practiced 2 of last 5 years as a community health nurse
High-risk perinatal nursing	0[a]	1500 hours of direct patient care in maternal and child health nursing practice Have provided at least 300 hours of direct nursing care in field for 2 of last 3 years (time spent in formal program for advanced study may count for 1 year) Have 30 contact hours of continuing education in field within last 3 years

[a]First examination was given in October 1982.
NOTE: Taken from American Nurses' Association. *1933 Certification Catalog.* Kansas City, Mo.: American Nurses' Association, 1982.
Reprinted from Nursing and Nursing Education: Public Policies and Private Actions, with permission of the National Academy Press, Washington, DC, 1983.

Title of Specialty Area	Total Number Certified	Eligibility Requirements for Certification
Maternal and Child Health (MCH) nursing	0[a]	2100 hours of direct patient care in MCH nursing 30 contact hours of continuing education in field within last 3 years
Pediatric nurse practitioner	450	Completed program of study that meets criteria identified by ANA and American Academy of Pediatrics in "Guidelines on Short-term Continuing Education Programs for Pediatric Nurse Associates" or "Guidelines for Nurse Practitioner Training Programs"
School nurse practitioner	272	Completed formal education program affiliated with an institution of higher learning of at least 9 months or 1 academic year of full-time study, including didactic and clinical components as outlined in the "Certification Guidelines for Educational Preparation of School Nurse Practitioners"
Adult nurse practitioner	2468	Completed formal educational program affiliated with institution of higher learning of at least 9 months or 1 academic year of full-time study including didactic and clinical components as outlined in the "Certification Guidelines for Educational Preparation of Adult Nurse Practitioners"
Family nurse practitioner	2630	Completed formal educational program affiliated with an institution of higher learning of at least 9 months or 1 academic year of full-time study, including didactic and clinical components as outlined in "Certification Guidelines for Educational Preparation of Family Nurse Practitioners"
Gerontological nurse practitioner	91	Completed formal program of study that prepares nurses to function as adult, family, or gerontologic nurse practitioners as outlined in "Guidelines for Nurse Practitioner Training Programs"

TABLE 3   Nurses' Association of the American College of Obstetrics and Gynecology (NAACOG) Specialty Certification

Title of Specialty Area	Total Number Certified	Eligibility Requirements for Certification
Inpatient obstetric nurse	865	2 years of experience in field Employment in field within last 2 years
Neonatal intensive care nurse	405	2 years of experience in field Employment in field within last 2 years
Neonatal nurse clinician/practitioner	0[a]	2 years of experience in field or certification as an NICU nurse Graduation from neonatal nurse clinician/practitioner program that is at least 12 weeks long and acceptable to NAACOG, or 4 years of RN employment in NICU with at least 2 years as a neonatal nurse practitioner or clinician
OB/GYN nurse practitioner	2284	Completion of formal nurse practitioner program that has at least 3 months of OB/GYN content, is at least 12 weeks in length, and is found acceptable to NAACOG
Maternal, gynecologic, and neonatal nursing (joint certification with ANA)	414	No longer offered

[a]First examination was offered in 1983.
Reprinted from Nursing and Nursing Education: Public Policies and Private Actions, with permission of the National Academy Press, Washington, DC, 1983.

7 Knowing Trends

BARBARA O. McGETTIGAN

The popularity of science fiction computer games, space war films, and trends books points to an interest in, if not an obsession with, the future. Futurology is an emerging field with a rising status as an academic discipline. Over 400 colleges and approximately 12 think tanks in the business setting currently are developing strategies and programs to predict the future (Wellborn, 1980). Government agencies and major industries increasingly employ house futurists. This surging interest has carried over into the health care field; hospitals are expanding their efforts to explore the future and project trends.

Emphasis on the future originates from recognizing the rapid pace of change and realizing that we must plan for imminent tomorrows. Furthermore, we shape a preferred future by our visions and plans for realizing it.

In Chapter 6 you formulated several possible professional goals that dovetailed with personal goals. Now you will investigate the influence of the future on these goals and evaluate the plausibility of your possible career paths. A sense of the directions of society, health, and nursing helps you plan to reach a career goal. Visions and projections of the future can confirm the lasting nature of one career path or predict the obsolescence of another.

If, for example, one of your personal career goals is related to work with children, it would be important for you to know if the younger population in your area was decreasing. The decrease in population might subsequently decrease the demand for child health care and pediatric nursing. You would then modify your career goal to work with a different age group, or to relocate your practice where the need for pediatric nursing would be greater. If your planned nursing focus was highway safety, a projection that microcomputer sensing devices would reduce car accidents to 40% of current levels would make you reconsider your career goal and plan.

If your career goal is coronary care nursing, being aware of the projected incidence and prevalence of cardiovascular disease, societal behaviors related to risk factors, and projected technology and scientific capabilities could modify aspects of your career goal and plan. Changes in lifestyle, exercise, diet and stress management, technologic advances in remote monitoring, anticipated medical discoveries of cause and treatment of arteriosclerosis, along with the current decline in mortality rates from heart disease depict a long-term trend of diminishing use of coronary care units. Of course, the impact in any one locale will vary by factors such as the population profile and the current nature of health care facilities. By identifying and considering relevant trends, however, you might maintain a coronary care focus, expand it to include health education, or change your setting from a coronary care unit to the community.

In establishing, modifying, and planning career directions, you need to appraise consistently the impact of the future. To implement a goal of teaching nursing at the university level, you should consider, for instance, the proliferation of home computers, the potential of satellite telecommunication, effects of language barriers in a multinational society, and the growing demand for nurses with doctorate degrees in academia. Career plans may include learning about computer programming and video, plotting methods and time frames for doctoral preparation, and gaining exposure to students of various ethnicities in travel–study tours.

If you manage a career with an appreciation of trends and an awareness of the future, you can be proactive rather than reactive, rooted in reality rather than the ideal, and cope more effectively and comfortably with uncertainty. But if you ignore trends and projections, you will suffer the consequences of unanticipated changes. Without consideration for changing professional expectations, growing obsolescence of a particular nursing role, or expanding and new consumer demands, you may be left without career requirements, directions, or opportunity. This can evoke feelings of anger, isolation, frustration, and grief.

By anticipating what the future will bring, you learn how to respond. The more outcomes and events can be anticipated, the more impact on a career can be projected, and the more influences can be predicted, the better prepared you will be to cope effectively with the future as it unfolds. Considering the future as it relates to your career is like rehearsing for a play. You learn how to act in the future the way you practice the scenes and lines for a role. The more elaborately you imagine and play out your lines, the greater the likelihood of a stunning opening night performance. Just like unanticipated life events, cues can be missed or props mislaid, but having rehearsed, you adapt to modifications or unusual situations with greater aplomb.

To anticipate the future, you need to decide what you will include in your perspective and the methods you will use to arrive at a vision of tomorrow. What to include in your perspective and the indicators that depict what is going on in these areas are described in the next section. You decide which parameters are most relevant for your career goal. Methods for future forecasting are presented in exercises, giving you an opportunity to apply sample forecasts to your professional goals.

Areas and Indicators of Change

Nursing career planners need to consider societal, health, and nursing issues. In each of these areas are key indicators of events and changes that delineate trends and outcomes. These three parameters and their indices are considered here to emphasize that what happens in nursing affects and is affected by the health care field and by society.

Societal Change

Future events and changes in society can be anticipated by assessing demographics, organizational styles, and technologic, economic, and political directions (Hunt, 1981).

Demographics. The current pattern and projected changes in age, location, and ethnicity of the population are key societal parameters. What are the projected percentages of the population that will be young, middle-aged, over age 65, or 75 years and older? Projections on percentages of the population 65 years and older are shown in Figure 7–1. Is the population rapidly growing at, for instance, 2% per year, or are couples deferring childbearing, slowing the rate of growth to 0.5% per year? What is the average life expectancy and median age? What is the percent of households with single persons or parents? Where is the population moving geographically? Are there controls and regulations that directly or indirectly affect urbanization? Will there be dense, inner-city crowding or incentives for rural location and relief of urban sprawl? Consider the ethnicity and rate of population growth along with the degree of subculture integration. Are subcultures actively integrated into the dominant culture, or is there simply tolerance with powerless minority groups? Major sources of data are the Bureau of the Census, Department of Commerce, the National Center for Health Statistics, and the Social Security Administration.

Population age, growth, location, movement, and ethnicity apply in various ways to career planning. For instance, the geographic location of people indicates where jobs will be. The age of clientele can be projected from population shifts. The health needs and thus the focus of practice will vary with the age, sex, and ethnicity of client populations. Population densities are indicators of what psychosocial, communicable, and ecologic health problems can be expected.

Figure 7–1 Number of elderly by age groups in the
United States: 1950–2050.

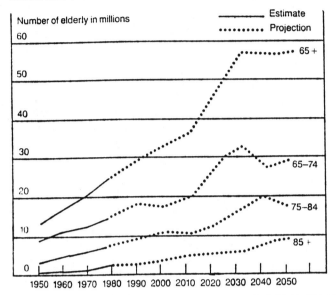

From US Bureau of the Census, Current Population Reports, Series P–25, No. 764, US GPO, Washington, DC, 1977.

Organizational Style. The manner in which groups of people assign and discharge authority and responsibility provides clues about the way people in society will interact with health care professionals and the health care delivery system. The types of health care interventions that are going to be valued may be ascertained by assessing this trend. For instance, interest in and demand for health education and self-care may reflect a more participatory organization profile than would demands for surgery or hospitalization. The way health care agencies are organized will generally reflect societal organizational styles. The role of the professional nurse and the role of nurse managers in particular will reflect the way this organizational style trend evolves. Hospital reports, organizational charts, the general literature, and your observations are important data sources on organizational style.

Technology. Trends in technology, the application of science to industry and commerce, can be discerned by asking where and at what speed advances are occurring and being forecast. You can analyze technology and technologic advances by exploring what is happening with energy, farming and food, building, housing, telecommunications, and transportation. These technologies may be incorporated in some ways by the health care industry. Identify the current and projected purpose or emphasis for the application of technology. Will the emphasis be mainly to increase and diversify production, to protect the environment, to regulate or improve personal or interpersonal behavior, or all of these? How rapidly will technologic advances take place? One indicator of the speed of advance is the relative amount of funding in various major companies for research and development. Business and economic journals such as *Forbes* publish annual directories of the largest businesses, showing industrial successes, trends, and types of expenditures, including research and development.

The types, purpose, and speed of technologic advances have much relevance to your career planning and ongoing assessment of goals. For example, types of health problems can be affected greatly by the degree of environmental protection. A trend toward the use of technology for protecting the environment could influence the focus and location of nursing care providers. On the other hand a trend away from environmental protection, such as increased use of fertilizers, can result in hazards, toxins, and health problems, which influence your nursing focus. The production of goods in space and advances in electrically powered vehicles could significantly reduce air pollution and markedly decrease lung cancer morbidity and mortality rates. If you have a career goal of pulmonary nursing you should consider options and anticipate the impact of such technologic advances.

It is important to be cognizant of technologic advances that can directly affect health care. Improved wound healing with electronically stimulated dressings could affect the skin-care or surgical-care specialist. Technologic advances in nerve regeneration could markedly alter care for those with spinal cord injuries. Likewise, genetic engineering could have significant impact on the job of a nurse caring for babies with congenital defects or of a nurse dealing with cancer victims.

The Economy.   The growth and stance of the economy both nationally and internationally are important trends to track. Indices include the stock market, the Gross National Product (GNP), the Consumer Price Index, inflation and interest rates, income levels, employment rates, and hiring expectations. Is the general economy prosperous, with an average annual growth rate of the GNP at 5% or more, or is it depressed below 0.5%? Are interest rates rising or falling? Are incomes stable or fluctuating and who is affected? How sound economically is the country overall as well as particular companies or groups of industries? What are projections of government spending and the deficit? Sources of information include business journals such as the *Wall Street Journal* or *Business Week*, the economic census, stock exchanges, and brokerage house reports. Federal Reserve bulletins and large bank letters on international and state economics often are available free.

The state of the economy influences the health care system, technologic advances, and nursing services. The general economy will influence the money available for capital expenses, program expansion, and personnel hiring. When prosperous, consumers may have more money available to supplement employers' coverage of medical care or health promotion services. Industries may be able to pay for full employee health coverage as a result of prosperity. In times of a depressed economy, neither the consumer nor the employer is able to cover all basic services and cannot consider specialized or elective services.

The state of the economy influences the general structure and ownership of the health care system, the supply of health care professionals, and the availability of jobs. It can influence the types of health problems, especially those related to violence and stress. Personal income is among the factors that affect general health and infant mortality rates.

The general state of the economy can also give clues as to when to propose new client services or make changes in career status. For instance, in a depressed economy with soaring insurance rates, programs for health maintenance that could show cost savings in lower health insurance rates might be attractive to corporations. A nurse practitioner planning to establish an independent practice would certainly assess the economic situation to see that enough money will be available for clients to pay for services that may not be reimbursed by selected payer sources.

The economic system can emphasize private expansion, government expansion, or some combination of both. Emphasis on private expansion results in concomitant expansion of and competition within private health care agencies. Conversely, emphasis on government expansion results in government dominating control of health care agencies. The control of health care influences many aspects, including the location of jobs, types of services, and philosophy of management.

Politics. It is helpful to be aware of the priorities of the federal and state government. Is the government emphasizing competition with cost containment and deregulation or expanding social and regulatory roles? The overall political priority of regulation or deregulation affects licensure (for example, individual versus institutional licensure) and scope of external monitoring on health care facilities and industrial health hazards. When the major government role is perceived as military buildup for citizen protection, money may not be allocated or available for housing, human development and education, or health. Establishing health care centers and availability of money for special needs would have low priority in such an environment as would money allocated for nursing education. The number and effectiveness of nurses in government can affect salary, health allocation, and rights issues for all nurses. Nurses can form a network among politically active colleagues, join government relations committees, and keep track of political trends through state nursing organization newsletters.

Health System Changes

Identify current health problems and needs, health care services and delivery systems, health care technology, economics, and political priorities. This information and projections for each of these areas is important in your career planning.

Considering the diseases affecting the population can give clues to the areas receiving ongoing financial support, benefiting from research efforts, and requiring services. Over the last 40 years, heart disease has remained the number one killer, although mortality from cardiovascular disease has decreased in the last 10 years. Refer to Table 7–1 for the causes of death over the last 20 years. Research in cancer and cardiovascular disease receive large amounts of money from the National Institutes of Health and from private grants and foundations.

When considering career priorities look at the difference in mortality and morbidity by age and population groups. Recognizing that accidents are a leading cause of death in persons aged 5 to 24 years old may influence a pediatric nurse's career focus. It is also helpful to look at the causes of major health problems in society. Major factors causing health problems today are not necessarily affected by medical solutions or direct intervention. Many health problems are related to lifestyles and poor health habits such as smoking, faulty diets, lack of exercise, and use of alcohol and other drugs. As poor health habits are remedied, changes will occur in morbidity and mortality rates. An aging population will mean increased chronic illness and disability.

Assessing changes and trends in the health care delivery system can be done by considering hospitals, other health care agencies, and numbers and

TABLE 7–1   Age-adjusted Death Rates for Selected Causes of Death, Selected Years 1960–1982

Cause of Death	Year						
	1960	1965	1970	1975	1980	1981[a]	1982[a]
	Deaths per 100,000 Residents						
All causes	760.9	739.0	714.3	630.4	585.8	571.6	556.4
Diseases of heart	286.2	273.9	253.6	217.8	202.6	196.3	190.8
Cerebrovascular diseases	79.7	72.7	66.3	53.7	40.8	38.3	36.1
Malignant neoplasms	125.8	127.0	129.9	129.4	132.8	131.6	133.3
Respiratory system	19.2	23.0	28.4	32.1	36.4	37.0	37.7
Breast[b]	22.3	22.8	23.1	22.6	22.7	—	—
Pneumonia and influenza	28.0	23.5	22.1	16.4	12.9	12.8	11.3
Chronic liver disease and cirrhosis	10.5	12.1	14.7	13.7	12.2	11.5	10.4
Diabetes mellitus	13.6	13.4	14.1	11.4	10.1	9.9	9.2
Accidents and adverse effects	49.9	53.3	53.7	44.2	43.3	40.2	37.1
Motor vehicle accidents	22.5	26.5	27.4	21.0	22.9	21.9	19.5
Suicide	10.6	11.4	11.8	12.5	11.4	11.3	11.5
Homicide and legal intervention	5.2	6.2	9.1	10.4	10.8	10.3	9.7

[a]Provisional data.
[b]Female only.
National Center for Health Statistics: *Health, United States,* 1983, Public Health Service. Washington, DC, US Government Printing Office. (Data are based on the national vital registration system.)

types of health care professionals. Are the number, type, and revenues of hospitals increasing or decreasing? Are the number of beds increasing or decreasing? Is the occupancy rate and length of stay rising or falling? What percentage of health care workers are employed in hospitals? What types of specialty units are opening or closing? Who is selling and buying health care facilities? Other than hospitals, what kinds of agencies are increasing or decreasing? Are nursing home facilities proliferating? Are ambulatory care, outpatient departments, surgery centers, or community health centers becoming popular? What is the current status and projected growth of the home care industry? What other innovative facilities and approaches to delivering health care are on the horizon? Is there a health emphasis in other institutions such as industry and schools? Is the overall purpose of the system preventive or treatment oriented?

Sources of data on current statistics and projected trends for health care delivery systems are the American Hospital Association, with its annual survey of hospitals and their manpower, and the United States Public Health System (USPHS) office of long-term care, with studies of long-term care facilities. The American Medical Association, American Nurses' Association, and the National Center for Health Statistics are also valuable sources.

Appreciating trends in the health care system and emphasis on health in other systems or institutions can be a key determinant in adjusting your career goal. If you are interested in midwifery, for instance, it may be important to understand the projections for free-standing birth centers. If your career goal relates to the chronically ill older person, you need to determine what type of health care services, facilities, and personnel are and will be available to serve the geriatric client.

Broad technologic advances give insight into health care technology. Discover what technologic advances are projected in pharmaceuticals, biomedical instrumentation, and services. How will these alter the functions and role of the nurse? For instance, will there be instruments that will so alter self-monitoring capabilities that the need for nursing assessment will decrease? Will genetic advances mean that new drugs, enzymes, and enzyme inhibitors will be produced, tremendously decreasing or eradicating certain chronic illnesses or radically influencing the way we treat persons with these illnesses? Also, how will technology affect the management of services and resources? With the addition of tools such as computers for managing patient information, supplies, and staffing, how will the nurse's responsibility, role, and image change?

General economics have an impact on health care economics. It is important to identify total health care expenditures, percentage of personal income that is spent for health care, and the proportion of the GNP focused on health. Has the percentage spent for health care increased or decreased over the last several years? Figure 7–2 shows the trends for the past 10 years. Determining the amount of government and industry expenditure for health is also important. Growth in new payment and financing approaches, such as those in preferred provider organizations, physician and hospital ventures, and health

Figure 7–2   *Rising national health costs: 1972–1984.*

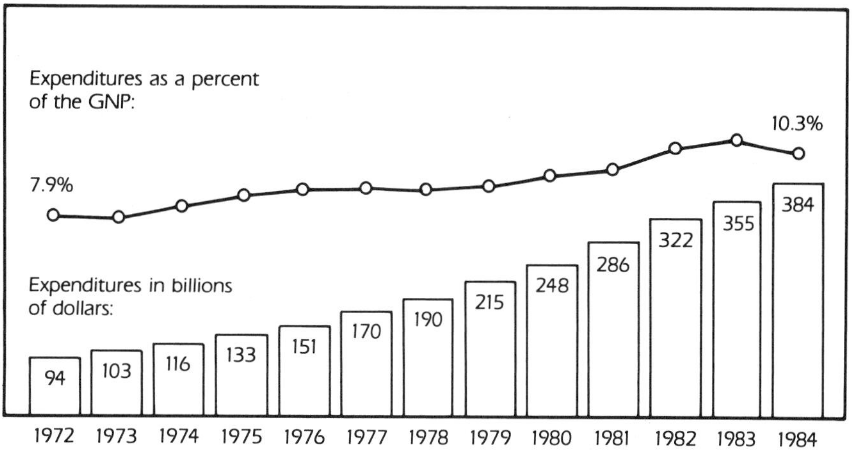

From Bureau of Data Management and Strategy, Health Care Financing Administration.

maintenance organizations, have resulted from rising health care expenses (Curtin, 1985). Since nurses represent the largest number of health care professionals and a significant budget item in hospitals, a tight economy in the health field can mean a shift in location and practice arrangements.

Health care planning priorities should also be followed. Depending on the strength of government's role in health and its allocation of money, government agencies may actively implement health care priorities. For instance, the Surgeon General's report on health promotion and disease prevention, *Healthy People* (USDHEW, 1979), lists five national goals and 15 principal strategies for health promotion and disease prevention to be realized by 1990. These statements on priorities are useful indicators of what will probably evolve over time, given available resources and lack of unforeseen events (Table 7–2).

A review of the health care system, major health problems, and priorities supplies important data for reality testing your professional goals, especially aspects of health focus and practice setting.

Nursing Trends

Trends of nursing practice, education, research, politics, and economics are extremely important to consider in establishing and evaluating a career goal. Consider what current statistics and projections tell about the type of practice in which nurses are engaged, the roles that they assume, and their geographic location. What are the shifts over the past 10 years in nurses working in hospitals, skilled nursing facilities, and home care agencies? Table 7–3 presents projected demands for nurses under three health system scenarios.

TABLE 7–2 National Goals and Strategies for Health Promotion and Disease Prevention

Five National Goals and Subgoals
1. A 35% reduction in infant mortality by 1990 to fewer than nine per 1000 live births. Subgoals: Reduce the number of low birth weight infants. Reduce the number of birth defects.
2. A 20% reduction in deaths of children aged 1 to 14 years, to fewer than 34/100,000. Subgoals: Reduce childhood accidents and injuries. Enhance childhood growth and development, and decrease special risks such as poor nutrition, child abuse or neglect, and learning disorders.
3. A 20% reduction of deaths among adolescents and young adults to age 24 to fewer than 93/100,000. Subgoals: Reduce fatal motor vehicle accidents. Reduce alcohol and drug misuse. Deal with problems of adolescent pregnancy, sexually transmissible diseases, mental illness, suicide and homicide.
4. A 25% reduction in deaths among the 25 to 64 age group to fewer than 400/100,000. Subgoals: Reduce heart attacks and strokes. Reduce deaths from cancer.
5. A major improvement in health mobility and independence for older people to be achieved largely by reducing by 20% the average number of days of illness among this age group. Subgoals: Increase the number of older adults who can function independently. Reduce premature deaths from influenza and pneumonia.

Fifteen Priority Activities to Attain These Goals		
Prevention	Protection	Promotion
Greater use of family planning services	Control of toxic agents	Smoking cessation
Improved care of pregnant women and newborn children	Implementation of occupational safety and health programs	Reducing misuse of alcohol and drugs
Immunization for vaccine-preventable disease	Accidental injury control	Improved nutrition
Control of sexually transmitted disease	Fluouridation	Exercise and fitness
Better blood pressure control	Infectious agent control	Stress control

Adapted from USDHEW, *Healthy People*. DHEW Pub. 79–55071, 1979.

What are the professional nursing organizations writing about standards for nursing practice, credential programs, and preparation for specific roles? Are expectations for education changing? What is the current and projected demand for and supply of nurses with various educational backgrounds? Table 7–4 portrays projected supply according to educational preparation needed by 1990. What are the current barriers and supports for education? What major developments are occurring in nursing theory and research? What kinds of

TABLE 7–3   Illustrations of Projected Demand for Registered Nurses (FTE) in Selected Practice Settings, December 1990, Under Three Sets of Assumptions

Practice Settings	Illustration I National Health Insurance	Illustration II Hospital Cost Containment	Illustration III Increased Ambulatory Care
Hospital (total)	1,024,000	906,000	844,000
Short-term hospital inpatient	799,700	688,100	653,000
ICU	(212,700)	(169,500)	(169,500)
Non-ICU inpatient	(569,800)	(501,300)	(466,600)
Nursing administration	(17,200)	(17,200)	(17,200)
Outpatient	111,400	104,400	77,900
Other hospital	113,000	113,000	113,000
Nursing home	100,000	100,000	100,000
Community health	123,000	123,000	123,000
Home care	30,000	30,000	62,000
Physicians' offices	64,000	64,000	22,000[a]
HMO-type organizations	10,000	10,000	32,000
Nursing education	57,000	52,000	50,000
Private duty and other	63,000	63,000	63,000
Total	1,472,000	1,348,000	1,298,000

NOTE: Detail may not add to totals owing to rounding off to nearest whole numbers.
[a]The sharp drop in nurse requirements in physicians' offices under Illustration III can be discounted; it appears to be only partially attributable to a shift in patient utilization due to increased HMO services. It may also be due, in part, to the fact that the existing model was not designed to accommodate such large increases in assumed HMO enrollments, which cause correspondingly large decreases in non-HMO physicians' offices. The resulting nurse requirements for this practice site may reflect the manner in which model components interact.
Reprinted from *Nursing and Nursing Education: Public Policies and Private Actions,* with permission of National Academy Press, Washington, DC, 1983, p. 58 & 73.

TABLE 7–4   Supply of Employed Registered Nurses, 1980 and Projected to 1990, by Highest Educational Preparation

Highest Educational Preparation	1980[a] Number	(%)	1990[b] Intermediate Projection Number	(%)
Diploma	645,500	50.7	614,000	35.9
Associate	256,200	20.2	475,000	27.8
Baccalaureate or higher	364,400	28.6	621,000	36.3
Unknown	6,800	0.5	—	—
Totals	1,272,900	100.0	1,710,000	100.0

[a]DHHS, HRA: The registered nurse population, an overview. In: *National Sample Survey of Registered Nurses, November 1980,* Table 3, p. 11.
[b]West MD: *Projected supply of registered nurses, 1990: Discussion and methodology,* Table 16.
Reprinted from Study of Nursing and Nursing Education Background Paper: Analysis of Career Differences Among Registered Nurses with Different Types of Nursing Education, with permission of the National Academy Press, Washington, DC, 1982.

curricula generally are available at baccalaureate, master's, and doctoral levels; what trends and clues are reflected in these curricula? Is the affiliation between service and education increasing or decreasing?

What are the priorities in academic and clinical nursing research? What kind of image and political force does nursing seem to exert? What are the numbers of nurses in local, state, and federal politics? What groups are affiliated with nursing organizations, and how powerful are they? How effective are nurses in lobbying for health issues, dollar allocations, and self-interest such as credential programs and equal pay?

Economics of nursing refer to current and projected salaries as well as the effect of diagnosis-related groups, reimbursement, and fees for nursing services. Nurse practitioners, nurse midwives, nurse entrepreneurs, and consultants should formulate, monitor, and anticipate changes in reimbursement related to independent status and use of services. Employed nurses should keep abreast of changing labor practices, strength of unions, and comparable worth issues, because these influence salaries and economic strength.

Key sources of data on nursing are *Nursing Outlook* for educational trends, *Nursing Economics* for fiscal issues, and publications of associations for political and social trends. Special studies and reports from the Institute of Medicine (1983), National Commission on Nursing (1983), regional boards, and the National Information Center, Division of Nursing (see resource guides in Chapter 4 Appendixes) add in-depth perspectives on nursing indicators.

Many factors should be assessed in developing a sense of the future. What is presented here is not exhaustive. There are numerous social, health, and nursing indicators that could be relevant to career planning. Ask yourself what facets of society, health, and nursing are most relevant for you. If, for example, your career goals involve surgery, you need to assess societal attitudes about—surgical or medical treatment, nontraditional healing or holism—that could support or constrain surgery. The growth or constraint of surgical treatment for major health problems and the overall increase or decrease in surgery relate to expected expansion and subspecialties for surgical nurses. The impact of technology on instruments and apparatus for surgery, artificial body parts, or organs must be investigated. The current and projected numbers of inpatient and outpatient surgical beds and surgical nurses will assist you in evaluating the expansion or contraction of opportunities.

If your career goal involves nursing education, you should assess projected preparation of nurses by position and service, professional recommendations for types and number of nursing programs, faculty–student ratios, and supply and demand projections for nurse educators in various programs. Additional trend areas to analyze for your career goal are societal values and practices related to education and projected technologic advances in educational delivery systems, demographic influences on age and culture of students, and public versus private support for formal education.

Exercise 7–1   Questions About the Future

Write a summary statement of your professional goals from Exercise 6–10 in
Chapter 6. Then place a check mark in the space provided next to those
indicators of change relevant to your professional goals. Finally, write specific
information that you need to appreciate the effect of the future on your goals.

I. Summary statement of my professional goals: _____

_____

_____

II.

Indicators of Change	*Specific information about the future relevant to my career goal*
A. Societal:	
_____ Demographics	_____
	_____
	_____
_____ Organizational style	_____
	_____
	_____
_____ Technology	_____
	_____
	_____
_____ Economy	_____
	_____
	_____
_____ Politics	_____
	_____
	_____
B. Health care system:	
_____ Health status	_____
	_____
	_____

_____ Health care delivery
     system

_____

_____

_____

_____ Economy

_____

_____

_____

_____Technology

_____

_____

_____

_____ Priorities

_____

_____

_____

C. Nursing

_____ Practice

_____

_____

_____

_____Settings

_____

_____

_____

_____ Research

_____

_____

_____

_____ Education

_____

_____

_____

_____ Politics and image

_____

_____

_____

Now that you have identified what you need to know about the future, the following section introduces you to some ways to get that information.

Methods

How can a vision of the future be obtained? What methods are used in forecasting? Prediction is certainly difficult and always risky; an art rather than a science. Both optimistic and pessimistic forecasts have proven inaccurate. Experts predicted at the New York World's Fair of 1939 that slums would disappear from American cities, and highways would be free of traffic jams. Others predicted in 1972 that we would deplete all our oil resources in 20 years (US NWR, 1983). We still have sufficient oil to fuel the automobiles that are still jamming the streets of our overcrowded cities.

Forecasting is further confounded by the unpredictable: volcano eruptions, plagues, earthquakes, nuclear accidents, catastrophes, and other upheavals that cannot be put into the scheme of forecasting. Regardless of the risks, attempts at forecasting are as ancient as the human race. Most simplistic and rudimentary are the use of crystal balls, soothsayers, or Ouija boards to decipher what the future holds. Although these divining tools can be secretly reassuring, truly helpful forecasting builds on knowledge and experience. Three major methods are useful in predicting the future: genius forecasting, Delphi technique, and trends projection (Stolovitch, 1979).

Genius Forecasting

Individuals such as Aldous Huxley from the past and Alvin Toffler of the present stand out as genius forecasters. Leaders in nursing who, based on their knowledge of the past, have the ability to visualize nursing's future include Styles, Jacox, Chaska, the Kalisches, and Mauksch. Forecasters tend to make their predictions at the ends of years and decades or for significant years such as Orwell's *1984*. Serious career planners need to consider the implication of futuristic insights. They also need to be alert to the innate human ability to follow the rhythms and patterns of events, to sense relationships and changes, and thereby predict and shape the nature of the future.

From daily contacts with consumers and direct experience with the health care delivery system and with other professionals, you undoubtedly have developed your own themes for nursing's future. For an opportunity to reach into your own forecasting genius before responding to the visions of others, complete Exercise 7–2.

Exercise 7–2 Your Forecasts for the Future

Imagine yourself in the year 2000. Take your time—settle your thoughts into your world of the future. What five newspaper headlines are you reading?

1. _____
2. _____
3. _____
4. _____
5. _____

What five headlines are you reading in the nursing literature?

1. _____
2. _____
3. _____
4. _____
5. _____

Given your forecast headlines, describe a day in your life in the year 2000.

_____

_____

_____

_____

In what ways does your vision of the future affect your current professional goals? Describe how your goals are supported or negated.

Goal 1: _____

_____

Goal 2: _____

_____

Goal 3: _____

_____

Exercise 7–3   Toffler's Forecasts

In his book *The Third Wave* (1980), Alvin Toffler envisions society moving toward a technologic era, following the industrial and agricultural eras. Third-wave diversity, decentralization, and concomitant need for information contrast with the uniformity and bureaucracy of a crashing industrial civilization. Although Toffler warns of the need to synthesize the various technical, social, and informational changes for a vision of the future, it seems helpful to look analytically at a succession of changes to develop a gestalt of the future.

Read the following sample of changes that Toffler foresees.

1. Variety of energy sources, with low and efficient use of energy in cars and other products, compared to single source and fuel wastes of the industrial era.

2. Smaller neighborhood work centers or work at home with computers and teleconferencing rather than commuting to big-city corporate offices and factories.

3. Regular space shuttles between earth and space, where advanced manufacturing and mining take place and space cities evolve.

4. Offshore housing and floating factories with aquafarming and aquamining.

5. Genetic engineering of new food and body chemicals.

6. Small television networks for communities of audiences that send programming, interacting with each other and with access to the essential resource—information.

7. The corporations that remain are decentralized with a greater degree of self-management and an emphasis on individual responsibility, adaptability, design capabilities, and resourcefulness compared to conformity, standards, and assembly-line values.

8. Variety of family and individual styles and roles with increased involvement of family. Home reemerges as central social unit, with an increasing role in education and caretaking of the elderly and infirm.

Given these aspects of Toffler's Third Wave, synthesize them into a statement that describes a vision of the future for you.

_____

_____

_____

What changes or effects does this vision of the future imply for you and your professional goals?

Goal 1: _____

_____

Goal 2: _____

_____

Goal 3: _____

_____

_____

Exercise 7–4   Jacox's Forecast

In an article, ''Address to the Next Generation,'' Jacox (1978) describes her vision of the year 2003. Read selected aspects of her vision provided here. For each item, write any implications it might have for your nursing career goal.

1. Between 25 and 30% of nurses are working in hospitals, while 50 to 60% are doing primary care, mostly in ambulatory care clinics. Some nurses work in extended care facilities; a few are on the fringe of the system.

    Implications for my nursing career goal: _____

    _____

    _____

2. Hospital nurses are mainly prepared in 2-year programs, while in primary care most nurses have baccalaureate degrees and approximately 25% have master degrees or above.

    Implications for my nursing career goal: _____

    _____

    _____

3. Nurses in hospitals engage in technologically sophisticated care of seriously ill people and are expected to know how to read and interpret a variety of complex monitoring equipment and receive instructions from computers. Hospital administrators, rather than nurses, perform personnel, budgeting, and evaluation functions. Nurses in primary care have greater responsibility for total patient care and also do patient teaching and health promotion as a major part of work.

    Implications for my nursing career goal: _____

    _____

    _____

4. You know the cause of most forms of cancer and how to prevent them. You also know that many diseases, formerly thought to be a natural accompaniment of aging such as coronary disease, stroke, and some forms of arthritis, can be largely avoided through preventive health practices.

Implications for my nursing career goal: _____

_____

_____

5.   Elderly persons are still given minimal care by poorly trained, poorly paid staffs.

Implications for my nursing career goal: _____

_____

_____

___

Exercise 7–5   Genius Forecasting in the Nursing Literature

Find four or five major nursing journals for the months of December or January of 1980 or 1985 (beginning decade or mid-decade). Browse through what the nursing geniuses, or recognized leaders, wrote about the future. Make a list of ten items that describe the future. Rank them according to priority by numbering from 1 to 10 in order of frequency found in the literature. Develop a synopsis for yourself of what the leaders in nursing are saying about the future. Describe what the nursing scene will be.

Priority   *Forecast*

_____   a. _____

_____   b. _____

_____   c. _____

_____   d. _____

_____   e. _____

_____   f. _____

_____   g. _____

_____   h. _____

_____   i. _____

_____   j. _____

Based on your rated list, write your view of the future nursing scene: _____

_____

_____

Summarize what your own and others' visions of the future mean to your professional nursing goals.

_____

_____

_____

_____

Delphi Technique

Another method for forecasting is the Delphi technique, first developed as a forecasting tool at the Rand Corporation. It is similar to genius forecasting but represents a collective genius, systematically eliciting what the future will bring. A series of questionnaires with feedback reflect group consensus on probable futures. Predictions about the future gleaned from the literature, from leaders, or otherwise hypothesized are listed and circulated to a large number of experts within a field. Each expert is asked to assign the probability for the occurrence of each listing by a specified future date. Personal predictions can be added to the list. The predictions, along with the group's probability ratings and any additional forecasts, are circulated two or three more times among the total group of experts. Statistical analyses of responses are made after each round and given as feedback for the next round.

Hill (1984) applied the Delphi method to nursing education administrators in the Midwest Alliance in Nursing. She sought insights about events in health care, nursing, nursing education, and specific skills needed to deal with anticipated events by 1992. Her findings indicate significant trends for nurses.

Health care
  Increased emphasis on integration of health maintenance into health care systems
  Increased demand for counselors in health maintenance
  Growth in competitive incentive programs for clients offered by all health care agencies

Nursing practice
  Use of computers by all nursing staff members for autonomous decision making concerning client care
  Use of highly skilled technical nurses for nearly all direct nursing care to hospitalized clients
  Use of technical and professional nurses according to uniform job descriptions for each ANA-organized category

Nursing education
  Faculty–student ratio in clinical experience to increase from the present 1:15

Managerial skills (needed by nursing education administrators to respond
to future predicted events)
    Computer language and usage; information systems knowledge
    Program analysis
    Trends analysis
    Coping with organizational complexity
    Monitoring student use of computer

The Delphi technique has been used in other ways in nursing. In 1981
Fellows of the American Academy of Nursing (FAAN) listed critical nursing-
related health care issues as priorities within the health care system. These
issues, comprising a 75-item questionnaire, were rated in three successive
rounds according to both importance to the profession and likelihood that the
academy could have an impact on the issues at a national level.

Exercise 7–6   Modified Delphi Technique

The results of the last round of the FAAN Delphi survey on the health care
priorities system (Lindeman, 1981) are summarized and listed here. Use this
list to do your own modified Delphi survey. Select four nurses whose
opinions about nursing are based on education or experience and circulate
the survey. Have each person, including yourself, read and anonymously rate
from 1 (highest probability) to 7 (lowest probability) the chance of this item
remaining a priority within 10 years. Tally the surveys after each round and
recirculate with feedback three times. Eliminate the highest and lowest score
on each item. Identify consensus items and compute the mean score of
remaining items. Indicate priorities found. Remember that low scores
designate higher priority.

Priority   *Items*

_____   a. Develop public awareness of the unique contribution nursing makes to
         health care.

_____   b. Improve public image of nursing.

_____   c. Create public acceptance of nursing as an independent profession.

_____   d. Ensure nursing autonomy through well-formulated nursing practice acts.

_____   e. Conduct nationwide research on the cost of nursing services delivered in
         strictly nursing models.

_____   f. Develop a large group of nurses who have developed effective skills in
         the political arena.

_____   g. Promote a strong role for private sector, third-party payers for funding
         nursing services.

_____ h. Clarify the scope and nature of nursing practice in primary, secondary, and tertiary care settings.

_____ i. Establish nursing as the primary provider in hospice-type care.

_____ j. Establish the baccalaureate degree in nursing as minimum educational level for professional nursing.

_____ k. Ensure a central work setting that enables real nursing care to be practiced and taught.

How can the priorities you found affect your nursing career now and in the future? _____

_____

By looking at these national issues from a local perspective, with the help of your local experts, you can more readily assess their influence on you in your nursing career.

Trends Projection

Trends projection relies on observing what is happening now and extending these events into the future. Trends are patterns that events depict rather than the events themselves. They depend on human judgment about the meaning of data from reliable, valid sources. Trends are general, not detailed, and are based on the present to project the future.

Perhaps the main drawback to trends projection is that events and situations rarely continue in a linear fashion. Swings and dips confuse the observer and make long-term patterns less than apparent. Periodic oil finds or new oil discovery methods can cause a temporary glut in oil resources; foreign embargos can lead to oil shortages. Restraint by users can weaken oil cartels, or adaptations in size and efficiency of cars can temporarily balance use of resources. All these events affect the pattern of the trend. Nonetheless, overall depletion of oil resources is a general evolving pattern, and methods of energy provision and use are needed to address this overall oil depletion trend. In like manner, the short-term increases in birthrate resulted from delayed childbearing by members of the baby-boom era. This phenomenon, however, is a temporary upswing in a segment of the population and should not be interpreted as a reversal of the long-term trend of an aging population.

In addition to problems of short-term fluctuations, trends cannot consider unexpected events. Who could have predicted the discovery of microbes or atomic fusion 25 years before these events occurred? Yet these events drastically and abruptly reshaped trends in health, welfare, and defense.

Trends cannot account for discontinuity between the present and the future. For instance, trend projections could not have described the civilization that emerged after the fall of Rome.

Various approaches to trends projections can be taken. For example, the Naisbitt Group (Naisbitt, 1982) monitors local events and behavior around the world. Using a method called content analysis, the subjects of newspaper articles are recorded as they are added or dropped, and notice is taken of their share of the available print space. The changes over time reflect actual concerns and interests of society and the general direction in which the country is moving. Naisbitt identifies five states that set trends: California, Florida, Washington, Colorado, and Connecticut. He suggests closely watching what is happening in Florida because its population profile now reflects what is projected for the entire United States population in 1995. Naisbitt's methods suggest to the career planner an astuteness in observing the emphasis and changes in the content of local newspapers and professional literature in projecting the fate of issues or new trends.

In nursing the Western Interstate Commission for Higher Education (WICHE) and the National Center For Higher Education Management Systems developed a model (Gray & Sauer, 1977; Elliott & Kearns, 1978) for manpower planning using mathematical formulas. By applying these formulas, both nursing supply and nursing requirements were projected for 1- to 10-year time frames. Essential to this approach were specific assumptions or estimates based on research and judgment of experts involved in the projection process. WICHE's model considered nursing requirements to meet "ideal" health goals and fulfill "recommended" staffing and educational criteria to address needs.

The Institute of Medicine (1983) used an historic approach, looking at actual past demands for services and projecting them into the future, allowing for demographic and health system changes. Historic trends were manipulated to demonstrate varying scenarios, "what if" situations, to show the impact of changes on the demand for nurses and on the health care system.

It is important to keep in mind that projections may use different models. Overall methods may be based on differing data, and may differ in basic assumptions. To become more familiar with the use of projected trends, complete Exercise 7–7.

Exercise 7–7   Trends and Their Implications

Review the list of general trend projections based on a review of key future resources: Naisbitt (1982), Institute of Medicine Study (1983), USNWR Special Report (1984), Coleman and associates (1984), Donley (1984), Curtin (1985), and ANA Cabinet on Nursing Research (1985). Assess and indicate the implications that you see for your professional goals. For each goal, place a check in the appropriate column next to each trend statement (+ indicates the trend supports the goal; − indicates the trend contradicts or constrains your goal; ? means you are not sure of implications and may need more information about the trend).

After rating the trends, add the number of +'s, −'s, and ?'s for each goal and place your totals in the spaces provided at the end of each column.

Trends	Goal 1 + − ?	Goal 2 + − ?	Goal 3 + − ?
Population			
Movement from the north to the south, sun belt population growth			
Limited population growth, longer life span with 15% of US population over 65 years of age			
Increasing number of women in the population			
Shrinking American family			
Rising single households			
Organizational style			
A change from hierarchies to networking, from centralization to decentralization			
A change from reliance on institutions to self-help for health education			
Gender and ethnicity			
Females on the move and at work			
Rise in the number and power of minorities			
Expected multilingual fluency, including English, Spanish, and computer language			
Equal pay and comparable worth to the forefront			
Technology			
Rapid change from an industrial to an information society, resulting in knowledge-based society			
High-touch experiences and environments such as hospice, birth and health centers, and home care to ameliorate high technology			
Proliferation of user-created computers, a robot population boom			
Pollution-free cars			
Rapid telecommunication promoting a world economy and psychologic networks			
Permanent base on the moon			

Trends	Goal 1 + − ?	Goal 2 + − ?	Goal 3 + − ?

General Economy

More money for recreation; a 24-hour-work week

Emphasis on growth and profit

Slowed rate of increase in health care but overall continued increase owing to aging and technology

Access of the entrepreneur to the economy owing to low capital outlays and value in brain power

Politics

Declining superpowers and increasing world peace owing to communication

Government under fire

Trend toward private enterprise, competition, and continuing cost containment

Business replacing politics

From federal to state regulation

Participatory rather than representative democracy

From political parties and unions to issues, multiple options, and individual packages

Health

Emphasis on early detection and treatment (eg, lasers to vaporize plaque in arteriosclerosis)

Major health care needs dominated by chronic diseases and disability

Health problems related to environment and lifestyle, including alcohol abuse, stress, and violence, receive increasing percentage of health care dollar

Heavy investment in wellness programs, employee health, individual responsibility for health, and demand for self-care strategies

Drugs to retard aging process and diet supplement for memory

Trends	Goal 1			Goal 2			Goal 3		
	+	−	?	+	−	?	+	−	?
Decline in hospital bed use, excessive malpractice expenses, major cost-cutting, and closure of many hospitals									
Growth of comprehensive health care supersystems or conglomerates									
Increase in "spare-part" medicine									
Genetic engineering; gene manipulation to cure inherited diseases and cancer									
Increased emphasis on primary care in HMOs, other arrangements such as preferred provider organizations									
Increase in nursing homes									
Rapid growth in ambulatory care and services in various accessible community neighborhood locations									
Dominant health care concerns including patient advocacy, ethical dilemma, and the right of access to health care									
Prospective payment system for all payer groups									
Complex health care monitoring and services									
Excess supply of MDs									
Nursing									
Use of computers for documentation, decision making, and patient care									
Need for highly skilled technical nurses, especially for hospitalized clients									
Increased collaboration with physicians and other health care professionals									
Increase in geriatric nurse practitioners									
Use of nurse practitioners for rural and inner city populations									
Focus of services on health promotion, illness prevention, and adaptation to chronic illness									

Trends	Goal 1 + − ?	Goal 2 + − ?	Goal 3 + − ?

Education
BSN as basic minimal requirement for entry into nursing practice

Increased expectation of master's and doctoral preparation for nurse administrators, managers, academicians, and specialized practitioners

Increase in competency-based education

Use of computers for instruction, management, and design of education

Shared roles between nursing education and nursing service with more formal affiliations

Research
Growth of government and private money available for nursing research

Increased demand for researchers in nursing service and all types of service agencies

Expanded numbers of nursing research centers in large university centers and free-standing think tanks

Professional politics
Escalated participation of nurses in local, state, and national politics

Strengthening image of nurses as trained professionals with a marketable product, due to media blitz

Economics of nursing
Sophisticated cost accounting for nursing service according to nursing diagnosis

Payment for independent RN and NP services reimbursable

Independent nurses contract with self-designed packages for services such as health education, patient education, nursing services, management services for HMOs, hospitals, and home care agencies

Trends	Goal 1			Goal 2			Goal 3		
	+	−	?	+	−	?	+	−	?
	Goal 1 totals			Goal 2 totals			Goal 3 totals		
	+	−	?	+	−	?	+	−	?

Case Example: Ellen

Ellen has the following thoughts after considering projections about trends. "Given one of my professional goals of being a school nurse for the public school system, working with grade school children, doing health screening and education to prevent physical and emotional problems, I see a slow population growth. There may be fewer children and even school closures. Also, money for the public sector is dwindling while that in the private sector is increasing. I could move, consider private school needs, or collaboration with groups of pediatricians to provide new health services to their clients on a part-time basis to supplement my part-time school nursing. Trends tell me I should consider getting an MSN and learning how to use computers in health screening. If research moneys are going to become more available, I want to strengthen skills and plan to conduct research in the school setting."

Case Example: Joe

Joe is very interested in working in a hospital with chronically ill persons and their families. Demographic and illness trends supported his overall focus. However, he started to think about the implications of smaller, possibly more stressed families with limited resources to respond to a chronically ill elder. Perhaps emphasizing group support for elders, use of robots, and computer networking for problem solving would become more important as persons try to assume responsibilities for self-care. Also, if hospitals decrease in number and accessibility, home or ambulatory settings might be a plausible and more viable career direction for Joe.

Case Example: Jane

> Jane, a nurse in staff development, reassessed her goals in light of trends. The emphasis on information and rapid change reiterated for her the necessity of her role in helping nurses access and apply new knowledge to nursing practice. However, the competitive and for-profit trends in the economy could be a negative influence unless she could show cost savings and revenue-generating efforts. Her new direction would emphasize alternate home study and computerized modules. With the projected need for baccalaureate and graduate education in nursing as well as the projected trend toward a generally aging population, she would expand her services to include career, retirement, and cross-training advisement. Jane's analysis of trends not only sparked ideas for programs and services, but gave her a vision of a potential new goal: consumer health education in community neighborhood locations.

Analyzing the effects of trends on nursing practice helps you shape or reshape your goals. You may reject one professional goal as highly improbable because few trends seem to support it. You may further refine or adapt other goals you were considering. You may validate one or two professional goals as being quite viable and on target with other futurists' projections. Broad professional goals become more probable career goals with trends analysis.

As you applied various sample visions or projections about the future in this chapter, you already may have narrowed your goals or changed ideas as to setting, role, or other practice dimensions. There may still be specific areas or indications of change that you need to investigate prior to reformulating your goals.

Exercise 7–8 provides you with an opportunity to rework your goals and list key assumptions about the future that will probably influence them. Making explicit assumptions about the future helps you track trends and goals. As trends change, you can make the necessary alterations in your goal or plan. If your vision of the future holds true, you will be able to actualize your career with an effective plan. Chapter 8 presents the final step in further narrowing professional goals, choosing one specific career goal, and designing a plan to reach that goal.

Exercise 7–8   *Writing Career Goals and Assumptions About the Future*

In the space provided rework your professional goals to reflect the trends you have analyzed. Then note the major assumptions about the future that influence each goal.

Goal 1: _____

_____

Goal 2: _____

_____

Goal 3: _____

_____

Assumptions about the future (list at least five)

1. _____

_____

2. _____

_____

3. _____

_____

4. _____

_____

5. _____

_____

References

ANA Cabinet on Nursing Research: *Directions for Nursing Research: Toward the 21st Century*. Kansas City, MO: American Nurses' Association, 1985.

Coleman J, Dayani E, Simms E: Nursing careers in the emerging systems. *Nurs Management* (Jan) 1984; 15(1): 14–22.

Curtin L: Where will all the money go? *Nurs Management* (Jan) 1985; 16(1): 7–9.

Donley R Sr: Nursing: 2000, an essay. *Image* 1984; 16(1): 4–6.

Elliott J, Kearns J (editors): *Analysis and Planning for Improved Distribution of Nursing Personnel and Services: Final Report*. US Government Printing Office, Human Manpower References, DHEW, Pub. # (HRA) 79–16, 1978.

Gray R, Sauer K: *Analysis and Planning for Improved Distribution of Nursing Personnel and Services, Nursing Resources and Requirements: A Guide for Statelevel*

Planning. Boulder, CO: Western Interstate Commission for Higher Education and the National Center for Higher Education Management Systems, Division of Nursing, Bureau of Health Manpower, DHEW, 1977.

Hill B: A delphi application: health care, practice, education and education administration, circa 1992. *Image* 1984; 16(1): 6–8.

Hunt R: Forecasting and planning strategies from now to 2010. Proceedings of a conference sponsored by BASHMET chapter of the American Society of Health Manpower Education and Training, AHA, November, 1981, Oakland, CA.

Hunt R: Social trends indicators. Class guidelines prepared for Future Studies course, San Jose State University, San Jose, CA: Ed. Instructional Technology, #276, 1981.

Institute of Medicine: *Nursing and Nursing Education: Public Policies and Private Actions.* Washington, DC: National Academy Press, 1983.

Jacox A: Address to the next generation. *Nursing Outlook* 1978; 26: 38–41.

Lindeman C: *Priorities in the Health Care System: A Delphi Survey,* pp. 43–44. Kansas City, MO: American Nurses' Association, 1981.

Naisbitt J: *Megatrends.* New York: Warner Books, 1982.

National Commission on Nursing: *Summary Report and Recommendations.* Chicago: The Hospital Research and Education Trust, 1983.

Stolovitch H: Four training activities to help you forecast the future. *Training/HRD.* (April) 1979; 61–65.

Ten Forces Reshaping America. *USNWR* (March) 1984; 96: 40–52.

Toffler A: *The Third Wave.* New York: Bantam, 1980.

US Department of Health, Education and Welfare: *Healthy People,* pp. IX–X; 21–145. US Government Printing Office, DHEW Pub. No. (PHS) 79–55071, 1979.

Wellborn S: What the next 20 years hold for you. *USNWR,* 1980; 89: 51–53

What the next 50 years will bring. *USNWR.* 1983; 94: A–Z.

8 Choosing Your Career Goal and Making Plans

FRANCES C. HENDERSON

In Chapters 5, 6, and 7 you established personal goals by assessing yourself, developed professional goals that are your preferred nursing options, and identified tentative career goals that evolved from your consideration of nursing, health care, and societal trends. Your next steps are choosing one career goal and developing a career plan for that goal. Choosing a career goal requires testing each of your tentative goals and weighing the outcomes. Your career plan makes your career goal operational, guides your implementation, and specifies how you will evaluate your progress.

A goal should be challenging enough to motivate you to realize your maximum potential for personal and professional growth, yet realistic enough to have a high probability for achievement. A challenging goal is one that you enjoy discussing with others; accomplishing such a goal yields satisfaction and fulfillment, and illuminates your career path for new goals and new opportunities. A realistic goal is one that provides measurable, observable evidence of achievement over a designated period of time. The time span of a goal should not be so short that it contributes little to life direction nor so long that it defies completion. In our rapidly changing society it is important to update and revise goals appropriately. This may mean setting short-range goals as steps along a long-term career path.

A six-step process for choosing your career goal and making your plan is illustrated in Figure 8–1. Specific guidelines and exercises are included in discussions of each step.

Figure 8–1 Six steps toward choosing your career goal and making a career plan.

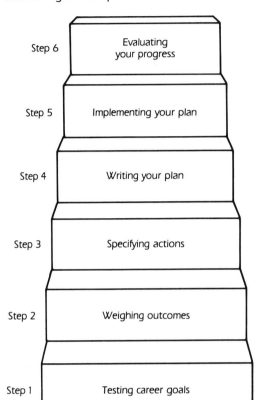

Step 6 — Evaluating your progress

Step 5 — Implementing your plan

Step 4 — Writing your plan

Step 3 — Specifying actions

Step 2 — Weighing outcomes

Step 1 — Testing career goals

Testing Your Goals

You refined your career goals at the end of Chapter 7. The next key step is reality testing to ascertain whether an identified career goal will help you express your values and achieve the kind of satisfaction you most want. Reality testing further relates the extent to which you can expect certain outcomes (Weiler, 1977). These outcomes refer to benefits, risks, trade-offs, and the reality of requirements, all of which will be helpful to you in making your career plans (Herr & Cramer, 1979). To subject your goal to a reality test, visualize it as a garment that you want to fit well. Is the fit between you and the goal too snug, too loose, too long or short, or does it fit you, your characteristics, potential, and values perfectly?

Strategies for reality testing your goal may be highly individual, simple, or complex. In addition to fitting your goal to your profile, other suggested reality testing strategies include informational interviewing, written resources, observing, and networking. The more information you collect about the realities of your goal and the better informed you are of possible outcomes, the better able you are to support the feasibility of your career direction.

Exercise 8–1   Testing the Fit of Your Career Goal

To test the fit of your goals, first refer to Exercise 7–8, and consider the congruence between each of your career goals, personal profile, preferred nursing options, and the trends most likely to affect it. Then respond to the following questions by identifying the extent to which you are satisfied with the results. Rank your responses on the scale provided by circling the appropriate number (0, not satisfied; 1, minimally satisfied; 2, satisfied; 3, highly satisfied).

1. To what extent are you satisfied with the consistency of personal traits, nursing options, and trends with your first career goal?

Career Goal 1	Not Satisfied	Minimally Satisfied	Satisfied	Highly Satisfied
Personal traits				
a. Needs	0	1	2	3
b. Values	0	1	2	3
c. Interests	0	1	2	3
d. Knowledge	0	1	2	3
e. Experience	0	1	2	3
f. Skills	0	1	2	3
g. Style	0	1	2	3
h. Stage	0	1	2	3
Nursing options				
i. Function	0	1	2	3
j. Role	0	1	2	3
k. Client	0	1	2	3
l. Focus	0	1	2	3
m. Setting	0	1	2	3
Trends				
n. Health care trends	0	1	2	3
o. Nursing trends	0	1	2	3
p. Societal trends	0	1	2	3

2.   To what extent are you satisfied with the consistency of personal traits, nursing options, and trends with your second career goal?

Career Goal 2	Not Satisfied	Minimally Satisfied	Satisfied	Highly Satisfied
Personal traits				
a. Needs	0	1	2	3
b. Values	0	1	2	3
c. Interests	0	1	2	3
d. Knowledge	0	1	2	3
e. Experience	0	1	2	3
f. Skills	0	1	2	3
g. Style	0	1	2	3
h. Stage	0	1	2	3
Nursing options				
i. Function	0	1	2	3
j. Role	0	1	2	3
k. Client	0	1	2	3
l. Focus	0	1	2	3
m. Setting	0	1	2	3
Trends				
n. Health care trends	0	1	2	3
o. Nursing trends	0	1	2	3
p. Societal trends	0	1	2	3

3.   To what extent are you satisfied with the consistency of personal traits, nursing options, and trends with your third career goal?

Career Goal 3	Not Satisfied	Minimally Satisfied	Satisfied	Highly Satisfied
Personal traits				
a. Needs	0	1	2	3
b. Values	0	1	2	3
c. Interests	0	1	2	3
d. Knowledge	0	1	2	3
e. Experience	0	1	2	3
f. Skills	0	1	2	3
g. Style	0	1	2	3
h. Stage	0	1	2	3

Career Goal 1	Not Satisfied	Minimally Satisfied	Satisfied	Highly Satisfied
Nursing options				
i. Function	0	1	2	3
j. Role	0	1	2	3
k. Client	0	1	2	3
l. Focus	0	1	2	3
m. Setting	0	1	2	3
Trends				
n. Health care trends	0	1	2	3
o. Nursing trends	0	1	2	3
p. Societal trends	0	1	2	3

Scoring

There are 16 test items for each goal. Add your ratings for each goal to obtain your score. The maximum score for each item is three, therefore a score of 48 indicates you are highly satisfied with the fit of your goals.

Use this chart to record your test results for each of your career goals. If you changed the ranking order of your goals based on your test results, record the revised order in the column provided.

Goal	Score	Revised Order of Goals
1		
2		
3		

Informational Interviewing

Informational interviewing is another reality testing approach (Bradley, 1983). This strategy helps you assess from others' specific input how realistic your goal is, the requirements, extent of satisfaction, extrinsic rewards, and potential risks and losses. Exercise 8–2 includes questions you might ask three persons involved in the practice you indicated as your goal (McGettigan, 1982).

Exercise 8–2   Interview Questions and Findings

I.   Description of practice or position

    a. What exactly do you do?

       1. _____

       2. _____

       3. _____

    b. With what population do you work?

       1. _____

       2. _____

       3. _____

    c. What are the client problems or phenomena that you encounter?

       1. _____

       2. _____

       3. _____

    d. What knowledge and skills do you use most?

       1. _____

       2. _____

       3. _____

II. Requirements

    a. What is the minimum educational preparation for this position or practice?

       1. _____

       2. _____

       3. _____

    b. What special preparation or experience is required?

       1. _____

       2. _____

       3. _____

III. Satisfaction

    a. What do you like *best* about your position or practice?

       1. _____

       2. _____

3. _____

b. What do you like *least* about it?

1. _____

2. _____

3. _____

c. What are the intrinsic rewards you experience (eg, sense of accomplishment, contribution, meaningfulness)?

1. _____

2. _____

3. _____

d. What are the extrinsic rewards that are most significant to you (eg, salary, work schedule, opportunities for advancement)?

1. _____

2. _____

3. _____

IV. Risks and losses

a. What risks are involved (eg, overload, underload, job security)?

1. _____

2. _____

3. _____

b. What losses are involved (eg, lost skills, time constraints, diminished resources)?

1. _____

2. _____

3. _____

Researching Print Media

One approach to researching print media to determine the realism of your career goals is to select at least three current articles from appropriate publications. After you read each one, make a note of what is stated about the practice that is significant for you and your goal. Ask yourself whether it does or does not support your expectations. In Exercise 8–3 record the articles selected and indicate the extent to which they supported your career goal by circling Yes or No.

Exercise 8—3   Print Media Test

	Goal	Key articles	Supports career goal?

1. a. _____   Yes   No

   _____

   _____

   b. _____   Yes   No

   _____

   _____

   c. _____   Yes   No

   _____

   _____

2. a. _____   Yes   No

   _____

   _____

   b. _____   Yes   No

   _____

   _____

   c. _____   Yes   No

   _____

   _____

3. a. _____   Yes   No

   _____

   _____

   b. _____   Yes   No

   _____

   _____

   c. _____   Yes   No

   _____

   _____

Observing and Networking

You can answer some of the questions listed in Exercise 8–2 by observing persons involved in the practice commensurate with your goals. Your observations will enhance, validate, or refute the responses of those whom you interviewed. Likewise, you can use your networking opportunities to glean input about specific aspects of your career goal that support or augment previous input or expectations.

Exercise 8–4 Summarizing Test Results

Consider each of your goals separately, using your results from previous exercises in this chapter to rate the extent of realism in your goals. Circle the appropriate number for each item in the three sections (0, unrealistic; 1, minimally realistic; 2, realistic; 3, highly realistic).

Goal testing method	Unrealistic	Minimally realistic	Realistic	Highly realistic
A.	0	1	2	3
Informational interview	0	1	2	3
Print media	0	1	2	3
Observation	0	1	2	3
Networking	0	1	2	3
B.	0	1	2	3
Informational interview	0	1	2	3
Print media	0	1	2	3
Observation	0	1	2	3
Networking	0	1	2	3
C.	0	1	2	3
Informational interview	0	1	2	3
Print media	0	1	2	3
Observation	0	1	2	3
Networking	0	1	2	2

Exercise 8–5 Weighing the Outcomes of Each Career Goal

Five questions have been designed to help you weigh the outcomes of each of your career goals. For each question, consider the probability of occurrence on a scale of 0 to 100%. Record your estimated probability for each goal and divide each sum by 5. Record your final score in the appropriate space at the end of each column.

Outcome questions	Goal A probability (%)	Goal B probability (%)	Goal C probability (%)
1. To what extent is it likely that this practice or position is a reality for you?			
2. How likely is it that you have or will meet the requirements for this position?			
3. How likely is it that this position or practice will satisfy you?			
4. To what extent is it likely that you will avoid significant risks or losses associated with this choice?			
5. To what extent do you value this choice?			
Subtotal:	_____	_____	_____
Divide subtotal by 5 and round to nearest whole number:	_____	_____	_____
Revised ranking of goals based on weighing results:	_____	_____	_____

The following is a sample of a completed weighing exercise.

Outcome questions	Goal A probability (%)	Goal B probability (%)	Goal C probability (%)
1. To what extent is it likely that this practice or position is a reality for you?	90	70	99
2. How likely is it that you have or will meet the requirements for this position?	100	60	100
3. How likely is it that this position or practice will satisfy you?	98	50	99
4. To what extent is it likely that you will avoid significant risks or losses associated with this choice?	50	50	50
5. How greatly do you value this choice?	100	70	100
Subtotal:	438	300	448
Divide subtotal by 5 and round to nearest whole number:	88	60	90
Revised ranking of goals based on weighing results:	2	3	1

As a result of Exercise 8–5, you chose the one most important career goal for you at this time that also has the greatest probability of being developed into a viable career plan. You are now ready to specify your actions, which you will include on your written career plan.

Writing Your Plan with Specific Actions

Converting your goal into clearly specified actions and time frames is essential to the planning phase, making achievement of your goal a systematic and exciting process. As you look at your goal and the requirements needed to reach it, identify any areas that are lacking such as a special certificate, additional education or experience, or conducting a marketing survey for your own independent practice. Consider how you will fill any gaps, the actions you'll take, and by what point in time. A simple process of ranking your actions in priority order can be a helpful step in deciding what you should do first or what actions you can pursue simultaneously.

Career planning takes time. In fact, some may choose not to expend the energy or time necessary to do career planning. Dangers, however, lie in passivity. Unrealized dreams give rise to anger, anguish, and disappointment. Time spent in planning leads to the satisfaction of dreams made real.

A career plan can be written using any one of several formats. One example is a self-contract that includes an objective, a predicted positive outcome, a duration of time, a self-reward, and a penalty to be administered should you fail to meet your objective (Hagberg & Leider, 1982). A contract using the same format may be developed and entered into with a partner (Baldi, 1980). Three formats for writing your career plan are presented here. One format guides you through 12 components, which are designed to help you shape your plan as you design it (Exercise 8–6). Another is a one-page, open-ended format that can be used to summarize key components quickly (Exercise 8–7). Because your career plan may be one for career renewal, a format for a career renewal proposal is also included (Exercise 8–8). Select the written format you most prefer by looking at the referenced exercises and deciding which format or combination of formats you want to complete.

Exercise 8–6   Specifying the Components of Your Plan

Twelve components of a career development plan are listed here. Space is provided for your responses to questions related to each component. As you complete this exercise, you will begin to design a career path.

1. Goal: What do you want to do?

   _____

   _____

   _____

2. Rationale: Why? What is your motivation for this goal?

   _____

   _____

   _____

3. Involvement: State your willingness to devote time, effort, and energy to make this goal a reality.

   _____

   _____

   _____

4. Congruence: To what extent is this goal compatible with your personal and professional goals?

   _____

   _____

   _____

5. Time: By what specific point in time do you expect to achieve it?

   _____

6. Individual attributes: List your unique professional characteristics, knowledge, skill, and experience related to this goal.

   _____

   _____

   _____

   _____

   _____

7. Potential intrinsic rewards: To what extent will achieving this goal satisfy you in terms of a sense of accomplishment or achievement, happiness, confidence, or security?

   _____

   _____

   _____

8. Potential extrinsic rewards: What are the tangible rewards of your achievement of this goal (eg, monetary remuneration, medical, vacation, or other benefits)?

   _____

   _____

   _____

9. Requirements: List the specific qualifications necessary to meet the goal.

   _____

   _____

   _____

   _____

10. Your preparation: List the specific knowledge, skills, and other qualifications that you currently have related to the goal.

   _____

   _____

   _____

   _____

11. Additional preparation needed: Write the results of your comparison of items 9 and 10.

   _____

   _____

   _____

   _____

12. Objectives and actions: Identify and list the objectives along the path toward achievement of this goal. For each, list specific actions to be taken.

   _____

   _____

   _____

   _____

   _____

   _____

   _____

If your envisioned career plan is related to your current position and you prefer a shorter format you may prefer the approach in Exercise 8–7.

Exercise 8–7   *Career Action Plan Related to Current Position*

Transfer your career goal to the space provided in item 1. Use the results of your assessments from Chapters 5, 6, and 7 to complete the skills and knowledge areas. Specify potential obstacles and a reward for yourself for adhering to your plan. This format does not include a space for objectives, but does include space for abbreviated action steps and target dates. Finally, it requires your signature and the date you complete it. The signing date and the projected date of completion will be especially helpful to you in monitoring your progress and in periodically revising your plan.

1.   My career goal or goals (related to current position):

_____

_____

_____

_____

2.   Skills required:_____

_____

3.   Knowledge required:_____

_____

4.   Additional skills or knowledge I need to accomplish the goal:_____

_____

5.   Obstacles:_____

_____

6.   Reward: How will I reward my effort?_____

Action steps	*Target dates*
_____	_____
_____	_____
_____	_____
_____	_____

Date for completion of this plan: Signature:

_____   _____

                                            _____

                                            Today's date: _____

Exercise 8–8   Career Renewal Proposal

This format for writing your career plan may be more appropriate when your goal is to renew career vitality in your current position. The format includes space for your career goal, objectives, and skills required. It focuses on assessing the extent to which you are currently meeting your career goal and on specifying the areas needing change to align more closely activities associated with your current position with your goals. Space is designated for your action steps, target date, potential obstacles, reward, and penalty if you do not meet the terms of your self-contract.

Name _____ Date _____

Position/Title _____ Div/Dept _____

Career goal: _____

_____

Objectives: List the objectives derived from your career goal that relate to your current position.

_____

_____

_____

_____

_____

_____

_____

_____

_____

_____

Skills required: List the skills required to complete your current objectives. Circle those skills for which you feel you need further know-how to satisfactorily perform in your current position.

_____ _____ Comments:

_____ _____

_____ _____

_____ _____

_____ _____

Career goal: Look at your career goal statement. Underline those elements met by your current position. Circle those elements not being met by your current position.

Needs statement: Complete the following needs statement as it pertains to you: To increase my effectiveness and satisfaction in my current position, I need/want the following changes (eg, change in environment, focus, function, more challenge, more knowledge or experience).

	Change desired	*Action steps*	*Target dates*
1.	_____	_____	_____
2.	_____	_____	_____
3.	_____	_____	_____
4.	_____	_____	_____
5.	_____	_____	_____

Obstacles: What might get in the way?

_____

_____

_____

_____

Reward: How will I reward my efforts?

_____

_____

_____

_____

_____

Penalty: What if I don't finish my proposal?

_____

_____

Date for completion _____ Signature _____

Today's date _____

Implementing and Evaluating Your Plan

Assume a personal responsibility to follow your plan systematically and to communicate your objectives to others. If you are not achieving the results that you had anticipated, or if you realize that you want different results, revise your goal and retest it, or modify your actions based on newly acquired data. Persevere in face of setbacks until you achieve your specified actions and feel that you are making progress in reaching your selected career goal.

Evaluating your career plan helps you determine how realistic it is. It will help you pinpoint constraints and focus on ways to reconcile them. By evaluating your plan critically, you can identify strengths and flexibility and consider alternative approaches when appropriate.

Examine your progress in reaching your goals based on your scheduled time frame. Re-evaluate your progress when there are problems. If you find your actions are not achieving the outcomes you expect or your time frames are askew, reassess and make appropriate changes. The process is continual and ongoing. Evaluation stems from implementation and leads to a reassessment with new goals and plans.

Exercise 8–9   _Charting Your Time Line_

One approach to evaluating progress with your career plan over time is by designing your own time line chart. This exercise allows you to plot and track your goals and actions over a 5-year period using Table 8–1. On the chart is a space to write your goal. Draw an arrow from the goal to the point in time by which you will achieve it. Next, write the objectives and actions toward the goal in the spaces provided. Draw an arrow from each action to the point in time by which you will achieve it. In using your chart to plot progress, you may want to place a check mark or star beside each action once it is achieved. Remember to reward yourself for your achievements and to be flexible enough to redesign your path if you find your goals or actions are unrealistic.

TABLE 8–1 Timeline Chart for Goal and Objectives

	Year[a]			Year + 1			Year + 2			Year + 3			Year + 4		
	1/1	4/30	8/31	1/1	4/30	8/31	1/1	4/30	8/31	1/1	4/30	8/31	1/1	4/30	8/31
Goal															
Objective:															
Action															
Action															
Action															
Objective:															
Action															
Action															
Action															
Objective:															
Action															
Action															
Action															

[a]Year means this year; year + 1, next year; etc.

A Lifelong Guide

This chapter has guided you through a process for choosing one career goal and making a career plan. You are encouraged to continue this process to determine additional goals and to further design and refine your plan. Career planning as presented here allows for individual changes and changes in circumstance; it is one that can be used as a lifelong guide for professional growth.

References

Baldi, S. et al: *For Your Health: A Model for Self Care.* South Laguna, CA: Nurses Model Health, 1980:33, 45–7, 141.

Bradley J: How to interview for information. *Training/HRD,* 1983 (April); 59–62.

Hagberg J, Leider R: *The Inventurers.* Reading, MA: Addison-Wesley, 1982.

Herr E, Cramer S: *Career Guidance Through the Life Span.* Boston: Little Brown, 1979.

McGettigan B: Course syllabus for N151, Nursing Options and Trends. Department of Nursing, San Jose State University, 1982.

Weiler N: *Reality and Career Planning: A Guide for Personal Growth.* Reading, MA: Addison-Wesley, 1977.

9 Using Career Management Strategies

FRANCES C. HENDERSON

Career management strategies as illustrated in the framework (see Figure 3–1) are major threads supporting career goals and connecting information areas. In this chapter four career management strategies are discussed with guidelines and exercises to help you use them effectively. They are attending the self, negotiating, marketing, and networking.

Attending the Self

Attending others is a key strategy in nursing practice, but nurses rarely apply such attention to themselves. Attending the self requires the same diligence you apply in client care settings, the same holistic concept, and an increased practice of self-advocacy as an ongoing endeavor in managing your career. It includes self-assessment, self-awareness, assuming self-direction in career decisions, and holistic self-care. Many of these themes have already been discussed. Exercise 9–1 is a summative list of selected self-attending activities, where you can rate the extent to which you engage in them. Consider your current use of these behaviors in managing your career.

Exercise 9–1   Summarizing Self-Attending Behaviors

Read each of the following items carefully and rate how frequently you perform each one by writing the appropriate numbers in the spaces on the right (0, never; 1, rarely; 2, usually; 3, always). Then add the numbers for items a–n and o–r. Finally, add your two subtotals to obtain your score.

Self-attending behaviors	*Rating*
a. Identify and rank your own values	_____
b. Identify your interests	_____
c. Identify your needs	_____
d. Appraise your knowledge as a nurse	_____
e. Appraise your skills as a nurse	_____
f. Appraise your experience as a nurse	_____
g. Gather and assess information for a decision important to you	_____
h. Generate and consider alternatives for a decision important to you	_____
i. Formulate a plan of action to activate your important decisions based on your unique personal style	_____
j. Formulate a plan of action to activate your important decisions based on your developmental stage	_____
k. Act on your personal goals	_____
l. Act on your career goals	_____
m. Implement a plan of action related to decisions that are important to your career stage	_____
n. Objectively evaluate the outcomes of your plan	_____

_____ *Subtotal (Maximum score = 42)*

o. Reward yourself for your achievements	_____
p. Engage in self-renewing activities	_____
q. Engage in health promotion activities	_____
r. Cope effectively with stress	_____

_____ *Subtotal (Maximum score = 12)*

Total _____

Maximum score = 54

Interpretation

The first step to empowering yourself is assessing your potential. Items a–n refer to personal characteristics, attributes, style, and stage discussed in Chapter 5. The maximum score for these items is 42. If you completed all or most of the exercises in Chapter 5, or if self-assessment is an activity you engage in frequently, your score will range between 30 and 42. Scores below 30 indicate that you infrequently engage in these behaviors. Items o–r address self-attending behaviors associated with self-renewal, such as a hobby, recreational and relaxation activities, or spiritually enriching ones. Attention to your overall physical and emotional health, including how effectively you cope with stress, is a requisite for generating the personal power necessary for effective career management. The maximum total score for this exercise is 54; 36 is average; and 35 or less indicates that you seldom attend the self.

Stress and Coping

Numerous definitions of stress have been written. What they all have in common is the description of physical and emotional reactions to factors in one's life that are perceived as threatening or unpleasant. According to Selye (1978), stress is the nonspecific response of the body to any demand. Life itself is a perpetual process of adaptation to a variety of demands, including socioeconomic, bureaucratic, domestic, academic, environmental and occupational requirements. Responses to these demands include frustration, feeling overloaded, boredom, and depression. Frustration is usually caused by perceived inhibition of your responses, resulting in anger, apathy, or depression. Feeling overloaded results from demands in excess of your capacity to meet them. Proceed to Exercise 9–2, gleaned from the work of Girdano and Everly (1979).

Exercise 9–2   Your Perceptions of Demands Versus Your Capacity to Meet Them

---

Choose the most appropriate response from the multiple choices provided for each of the 10 statements below. Place the letter of your response in the spaces provided.

_____ .   1. How often do you find yourself with insufficient time to complete your work?
        (a) Almost always   (b) Very often
        (c) Seldom   (d) Never

_____   2. How often do you find yourself becoming confused and unable to think clearly because too many things are happening at once?
        (a) Almost always   (b) Very often
        (c) Seldom   (d) Never

_____ 3. How often do you wish you had help to get everything done?
(a) Almost always (b) Very often
(c) Seldom (d) Never

_____ 4. How often do you feel that people around you simply expect too much from you?
(a) Almost always (b) Very often
(c) Seldom (d) Never

_____ 5. How often do you feel overwhelmed by the demands placed on you?
(a) Almost always (b) Very often
(c) Seldom (d) Never

_____ 6. How often do you find your work infringing on your leisure hours?
(a) Almost always (b) Very often
(c) Seldom (d) Never

_____ 7. How often do you get depressed when you consider all the tasks that need your attention?
(a) Almost always (b) Very often
(c) Seldom (d) Never

_____ 8. How often do you see no end to the excessive demands placed on you?
(a) Almost always (b) Very often
(c) Seldom (d) Never

_____ 9. How often do you have to skip a meal so that you can get work completed?
(a) Almost always (b) Very often
(c) Seldom (d) Never

_____ 10. How often do you feel that you have too much responsibility?
(a) Almost always (b) Very often
(c) Seldom (d) Never

Scoring and Interpretation

The scoring key is provided in the following table. Write the number of a's, b's, c's, and d's you selected in the appropriate column space. Multiply your result by 4, 3, 2, or 1 as indicated to get your subtotal. Then add your subtotals to obtain your total score. The lowest possible score is 10; the highest possible score is 40. The higher your score, the greater your perception of demands in excess of your capacity to meet them.

Scoring Key

Response	Points		Your Number of Responses		Subtotal
a	4	×		=	
b	3	×		=	
c	2	×		=	
d	1	×		=	
			Your total		_____

This exercise is designed to assess the perception of feeling overloaded. According to Girdano and Everly (1979), "The four major factors which contribute to overload are time pressures, excessive responsibility or accountability, lack of support and/or excessive expectations from yourself and those around you."

If your perception of demands is high, examine which factors or combination of factors is contributing most to this imbalance between demand and capacity to respond. All the factors that contribute to the excessive demands of overload are prevalent in perceptions of occupational stress. Additionally, occupational stress may be due to a lack of clarity in the expectations regarding your roles and responsibilities (role ambiguity), conflicting demands, or overlapping responsibilities (role conflict). Occupational stress may result in dissatisfaction with your position, a sense of threat, or a sense of futility. Occupational stress also is experienced with physical symptoms, feelings of emotional detachment, dissatisfaction with work, decreased performance, and negative self-concept. Table 9–1 lists some examples (Smythe, 1984). You may want to place a circle around those that apply to you.

Conflicting beliefs, lack of clarity in beliefs, or a forced choice between values also can create stress. Examples include uncertainty about values, beliefs, and goals; contradictions between your values and your style of living; and contradictions between your beliefs about yourself and feedback from others (Tubesing, 1979). Tubesing also lists feeling out of step with your life rhythm as another source of stress. For example, have you ever felt like you were pulling when you should be pushing, or were struggling to win an uphill race? It may be that the degree of effort and energy you were expending was in excess of your capacity, simply because you were marching to a beat dissonant to your own personal rhythm. It just may be a point worth thinking about.

Coping Strategies

Although coping strategies are numerous, they involve one of three basic approaches: removing the stressor, removing yourself from the stressor, or developing effective adaptation techniques. Effective adaptation techniques range

TABLE 9–1 Examples of Symptoms Related to Occupational Stress

Physical stress-related symptoms
1. Chronic fatigue, exhaustion
2. Insomnia or frequent nightmares
3. Marked weight loss or gain
4. Increased anxiety or nervousness
5. Muscular tension (headaches, back pain, teeth clenching or grinding)
6. Increased use of alcohol/medication
7. Menstrual changes
8. Gastrointestinal disturbances (nausea, vomiting, diarrhea, constipation)
9. Frequent body aches and pain
10. Decreased sexual interest

Emotional detachment
1. Disliking or feeling annoyed with clients
2. Avoiding co-workers
3. Calling clients names or referring to them by diagnosis
4. Feeling apathetic, lacking interest
5. Feeling like you are just putting in time and "going through the motions"
6. Frequent sick days
7. Focusing attention on paper work, nonclient-related tasks
8. Wanting to be left alone and not bothered by anyone at work
9. Having marital or interpersonal discord
10. Avoiding talking with your clients or their families

Dissatisfaction with work and decreased job performance
1. Feeling work is meaningless
2. Reduced productivity
3. Negative about everything at work
4. Procrastination and forgetfulness
5. Disillusioned with profession
6. Hate job
7. Generalized irritability
8. Increased opposition to any change
9. Job accidents or frequent mistakes, omissions
10. Low frustration tolerance
11. Unduly critical of co-workers, organization
12. Working below your potential
13. Inability to concentrate or solve problems
14. Feeling as if your job is destroying your personal life

Negative self-concept
1. Questioning your own competence as a health professional
2. Feeling depressed (hopeless, helpless, sad)

3. Being unduly self-critical
4. Feeling overwhelmed (too much to do)
5. Feeling as if you have nothing to offer
6. Feeling responsible for your client not benefiting from care
7. Feeling worthless, incompetent, or stupid
8. Being less creative
9. Experiencing isolation or alienation from others
10. Feeling of lowered self-esteem

Adapted from Edelwich J. Bradsky A: *Burnout: Stages of Disillusionment in the Helping Professions*. New York: Human Sciences Press, 1980, with permission.

from highly internal strategies such as meditation and relaxation to an analytical approach. Potter (1980) refers to one analytical approach, PACE: Pinpoint, Analyze, Change and Evaluate. She calls these four steps for deprogramming and self-programming "a guide for self-observation and for directing the rate and direction of your change." Another approach is the use of positive verbalizations, which may be done individually or with the help of others.

The aim of effective coping is to acknowledge the unique repertoire of coping skills that you often use spontaneously, several times each day with little conscious effort. This acknowledgement positively reinforces your coping image of self and self-confidence in using skills most familiar to you in coping with other demands. In so doing, you enhance your personal resourcefulness.

Marketing

The term *marketing* used within a framework of career management for nurses may seem foreign. Becoming comfortable with its use in this context may require learning new information or looking at what you know from a different perspective; it may involve an openness to change or a shift in attitude. The results of this section suggest a psychomotor response, that is, actually marketing your attributes as a nurse applicable to your career goals.

Webster's Dictionary (1984) defines marketing as "The act of buying and selling in a market;" or as "all business activity involved in the moving of goods from the producer to the consumer, including selling, advertising, and packaging." *Market* is defined as "the opportunity to buy or supply goods or services." We most often equate goods with marketing for a price and services with wages or salary. However, the reality is that as a nurse, you possess a supply of particular knowledge, experience, and skills to meet specific socially significant needs or requirements. Remuneration in proportion to delivery of your services is most often realized in salary. In this context the consumers of nursing services are both the clients and the organizations that employ nurses. Marketing involves the ability to package your attributes with your personal qualities, nursing expertise, and an awareness of your style and stage to fulfill your social responsibility as a person and as a nurse.

So, how do you do it? Position applications, cover letters, resumes, and circumstances in your employment setting provide you with opportunities to develop specific yet different innovative packages of your qualifications. When appropriate, seize opportunities to highlight them in networking situations and in job interviews. Create opportunities to inform your present employer of what you have to offer, and demonstrate your expertise consistently through your job performance.

Your comprehensive portfolio, which you compiled in Chapter 5, can be used as a valuable resource since it includes a comprehensive review of your knowledge, experience, and skills. You can use it as a resource for writing your curriculum vita or resume and for requesting letters of recommendation.

Marketing Your Expertise

Effectively marketing your expertise involves writing letters of inquiry, submitting a resume or curriculum vitae (CV), and engaging in job interviews. An inquiry letter for a position may be your first step in marketing your expertise. Limit it to one concise, uncrowded page, in which you acknowledge the position announcement, briefly state your expertise in terms of the advertised needs of the employer, and indicate your interest and availability for a follow-up interview (see samples in the Appendix at end of this chapter). An inquiry letter also may be written to inform a potential employer of your interest in specific positions in that organization. Because you possess varied expertise and employer needs and requirements vary, it is imperative that you prepare a resume or curriculum vitae to reflect the specifics for a given position.

Exercise 9–3   Your Marketable Expertise and Career Goals

Refer to the two or three career goals you compiled in Chapter 6. In the space provided, list the expertise needed to reach each of your goals.

1.   Career goal: _____

 Your marketable expertise: _____

 _____

 _____

 _____

 _____

 _____

2.   Career goal: _____

    Your marketable expertise: _____

    _____

    _____

    _____

    _____

    _____

    _____

3.   Career goal: _____

    Your marketable expertise: _____

    _____

    _____

    _____

    _____

    _____

    _____

Completion of Exercise 9–3 will help specify your expertise concisely in inquiry letters, resumes, and application forms.

The Resume

A resume is a summation of your education and experiences most relevant to a specific occupational objective, compiled for the purpose of being invited for an interview. It should attract attention and stimulate action. Resume formats vary; examples include functional, chronologic, or creative resumes. A functional resume should include, after personal data, a statement of your occupational objective followed by a summary of your qualifications. In a chronologic resume simply list your current position, your education, experience, special accomplishments, and additional skills beginning with the most recent. In a creative resume you may want to combine both the functional and chronologic formats, developing a specific resume for specific occupational objectives. A sample of each format is located at the end of this chapter. Exercise 9–4 will help you appraise your existing or newly developed resume.

Exercise 9—4 Appraising Your Resume

Six criteria for appraising a resume are provided here, as adapted from Moorpark College Counseling (1979). Appraise your resume by checking yes or no to indicate whether or not it meets each criterion. Write any comments suggesting improvement in the column provided.

Item	*Yes/No*	*Comments for improvement*
1. Overall appearance: Does it say "Read me!"?		
2. Layout: Is it well typed with neat margins and no spelling errors?		
3. Action-oriented: Do sentences and phrases begin with action verbs?		
4. Accomplishments: Are your accomplishments and problem-solving skills emphasized?		
5. Relevance: Have you made the connection between the job desired and your qualifications?		
6. Bottom line: Does your resume represent you well enough to get you an interview?		

Your resume should present your expertise attractively and accurately. It should be neatly printed or typed. Six-page resumes that chronicle 15 years of continuing education courses tend to detract from the initial screening process rather than impress potential employers.

The Curriculum Vitae

The curriculum vitae is a formal and precise account of your scholarly achievements. It is used primarily in academic settings for the purpose of evaluating qualifications for academic appointments, promotion, tenure, or honors. The CV differs from the resume in format, purpose, and use. Although resume formats vary, the format of a CV is specific, including the following information: education, experience, honors, professional memberships, publications, and advanced preparation specific to the academic purpose for which you prepare it. A sample CV is located in the Appendix at the end of this chapter. Table 9–2 indicates the differences between resumes and CVs and highlights specifics to guide CV development. Exercise 9–5 will guide you in critiquing your CV.

Exercise 9–5   Critiquing Your Curriculum Vitae

Five criteria for critiquing your curriculum vitae are provided here. Appraise your CV by checking yes or no to indicate whether it meets each criterion. Write any comments suggesting improvement in the column provided.

Item	Yes/No	Comments for improvement
1. Appearance: Does it look academic?		
2. Format: Is the required content properly placed?		
3. Significance: Does it chronicle your important scholarly achievements and accomplishments?		
4. Relevance: Are your scholarly achievements appropriate for the purpose?		
5. Bottom line: Have you presented this data well enough to obtain an academic appointment, promotion, or honor?		

The following case examples illustrate the points in letters of recommendation and whether a CV or resume is the appropriate choice.

Case Example: Michelle

Michelle Yvette Boyd has a doctorate in education and administrative experience in a school of nursing. She has a functional area of teaching with a clinical focus in mental health nursing, as well as years of experience as a psychiatric liaison nurse for a large medical center. Michelle is qualified for as many

TABLE 9–2 Differences Between a Resume and a Curriculum Vitae

Content	Curriculum Vitae	Resume
Personal data	Restrict to full name without degrees Current position title, institution, location, address and phone number Home address and phone number	Name, follow with title abbreviations (RN, MS, or if doctorate is highest degree, PhD, DNSc, or EdD) Current position title(s) Home address and phone number RN License number and credentials, eg, Public Health, Nurse Practitioner, specialty, teaching (subject) Date of birth and marital status optional
Education	List in chronologic order your postsecondary school degrees with years, names of institutions, and fields of study Advanced education, if relevant, may be included in separate category at the end	List all schools attended since high school: years, names, location, degrees, and areas of study; include other courses, if specific to position, for which no degree earned
Experience	List month and year, beginning and ending, position or academic rank, institution and its location in chronologic order Advanced or special experiences may be included in chronology or after, especially if some overlap exists Also include information related to research such as your role as principal investigator, research fellowships, projects funded or awaiting funding	Same as CV or if a functional resume, may specify roles and responsibilities of position, eg, "planned and coordinated a new outpatient pediatric clinic for a 100-client census at Marshall Medical Center, Houston, Texas, 1/80–6/83"
Honors	List scholarships only if you are recent graduate List year and title of honorary awards or degrees	Same as CV
Professional memberships	List professional organizations of which you are currently a member; if you hold an office, list it, date of your tenure, and special interest group or committee if applicable	Same as CV May include civic organizations and others if specific to occupational objective
Publications	List *all* publications in chronologic order; if co-authored, list names of collaborators in order of authorship; if more than one publication in a given year, arrange alphabetically by title. Use a recognized citation format	Same as CV
Format	No title or date Upper right corner: home address and phone number in 3 lines; upper left corner: name, current position, title, institution, location, address, and telephone number	Title (centered), date (upper right corner) (Date is optional but suggested) May contain subtitle, demographic data or personal data, listed sequentially Special accomplishments and additional skills may be added as last category, especially if relevant to occupational objective Make a note at the end "References available upon request"

as five nursing options, including consultant, administrator, educator, researcher, or practitioner. In packaging her experience for the position of associate dean of allied health at a private college, she prepared a creative resume, emphasizing her administrative expertise and deemphasizing her experiences as a nurse practitioner. When she applied for a position as an assistant clinical professor for a university school of nursing, she prepared a CV, chronicling her scholarly achievements. (Samples of both are included in the Appendix at the end of this chapter.) Since the university also offered a joint appointment option, Michelle prepared a resume, emphasizing her clinical and educational skills and experiences.

Michelle was equally selective in her requests for letters of recommendation. For the associate dean position, she requested letters from her immediate superior in her last administrative position, from a peer administrator, and the college president. For the teaching position, she requested letters from her immediate superior in her psychiatric nurse practitioner position, the dean of instruction of the college where she previously taught nursing, and her doctoral advisor. She used her comprehensive portfolio as a resource from which to select data for her CV, the most relevant experiences for each resume, and recommendations.

Case Example: *Laura Ann*

Laura Ann Tripp is a graduate of an associate degree nursing program. She is about to complete her BSN and has had professional experience as a staff nurse and assistant unit coordinator. Her professional objective is to become a unit manager. Laura wrote a functional resume and a letter of inquiry regarding a position as a unit manager; she also wrote a thank you letter to the director of nursing. (Samples of both are included in the chapter Appendix.)

Use your comprehensive portfolio to help you select the most appropriate persons from whom to request letters of recommendation relevant to the position you desire. Choose person(s) whose knowledge of your performance will validate and amplify your expertise. When requesting a letter of recommendation, let the person know the nature of the position you are seeking. Be sure to send a note or call to acknowledge your appreciation for the letter. When possible, obtain a copy of the recommendation letter for your portfolio.

The Job Interview

The job interview is the next step in marketing yourself. As a nurse, you have no doubt experienced at least one. Having completed the series of exercises in this book, you are fully aware of what you have to offer. Key factors to a successful job interview are listed here, serving as helpful hints to validate or enhance your interview experiences.

A. Learn about the organization. If you do not already have sufficient information or a resource from which to obtain it, request it in your inquiry letter.
   1. Is it federal, state, county, or privately owned?
   2. What is its administrative structure?
   3. What is the philosophy of the organization?
   4. What is its status in the community?

B. Prepare for your interview in advance.
   1. Study the position description and note your expertise for each requirement.
   2. Anticipate questions and think through your answers. You can usually anticipate questions such as:
      a. What is your understanding of the responsibilities of this position?
      b. Tell me (us) about your previous experiences in (teaching, primary care . . .).
      c. What do you see as your strengths related to this position?
      d. What would you do if . . . ?

C. Visualize yourself as an expert at the interview, and allow yourself to experience positive feelings about it.

D. Dress according to the image you want to portray.

E. Know the location and how to get there and arrive punctually.

F. Listen actively to both spoken and nonverbal communication, remembering that the philosophy of the organization is mirrored by those who work there. Do they portray an image with which you want to be affiliated?

G. Respond thoughtfully and specifically to questions.
   1. If the question is complex, or if you need time to compose your answer,
      a. Ask the interviewer to restate the question.
      b. Say, "Give me a moment to think about my answer."
      c. Seek validation from your interviewer by asking "Did I answer your question thoroughly enough?"
   2. If you lack expertise in a specific area about which you are questioned, say so candidly. For example, "My experience in clinical research is limited; however, it is an area that interests me and one that I'd like to learn more about."
   3. Describe your expertise using terms such as *responsibility, contribution, accomplishment,* and *accountability.*

H. Prepare your own questions in advance. Most interviewers ask you if you have questions after theirs have been answered. Use this opportunity to learn more about the organization and the position expectations. For example:
   1. To whom would I report?

2. Who would report to me?

3. What are your expectations of the person in this position?

4. What is the salary?

5. Tell me how you envision a typical day in this position. (Request this only if it seems appropriate.)

6. Tell me about the type of person you are looking for to fill this position.

I. Be sure to let your interviewer know when, where, and how you can be contacted.

J. Critique your performance. After the interview, replay the interview like a tape through your mind. Ask yourself the following questions:

1. Did I present myself to my satisfaction? In what way?

2. How do I feel about being employed in this organization?

3. If I were to experience this interview again, what would I do differently? The same?

4. What questions did I anticipate accurately?

5. What happened that I didn't anticipate?

K. Send a brief letter to the individual you interviewed with (or lead person of the interview team) the day following the interview, acknowledging your appreciation for the opportunity. You may also briefly reaffirm your interest in the position if appropriate.

In addition to this self-review, you may want to "replay" the experience with a friend, mentor, role model, coach, or family member.

Being Interviewed by More Than One Person

Interviews are often conducted by screening committees, interdisciplinary teams, or other designated groups. One reason for the group approach is the need to comply with affirmative-action hiring policies, so that one or two members of an interview team usually meet the requirements for gender equity and ethnic equity or are functioning in a designated role as the institution's affirmative-action officer. Additionally, representatives of potential subordinates or peers and your prospective supervisor may be members of the team.

Candidates often feel intimidated by team interviews. The following tips may be helpful. First, team interviews are usually fairly structured. All members of the team usually have reviewed the position description, participated in the screening of applications, and selected the top candidates for interview. The team usually designates a leader, formulates and reviews questions, and decides who should ask specific questions and in what sequence. At times, the team member who knows least about the expected response will agree to ask the question, enabling those who are best able to appraise your answer to listen carefully. Conversely, the person best prepared in an area may wish to ask the question. Often the interview team leader asks the first and last questions.

Your skills in assessing individuals, their spoken and nonverbal behavior, your memory, and your listening skills are all challenged in a team interview. Look directly at the person who is asking you the question. As you listen to the question, think how to address your answer specifically to the questioner. This is where your memory will serve you well. Try to remember whether the person asking you the question is your prospective superior, the organization's affirmative-action officer, or a potential peer, since this will help you to specify your answer. One exercise that may help you remember is to think of your position in the setting in relation to your interviewers. As they introduce themselves or are introduced, note the sequence, by order seated in relation to you, or by hierarchical position. Then visualize whether the person on your right, left, or facing you is the most senior member and where in relation to this member the others are seated.

Most interviews begin with a general question. Test yourself by determining who asked it of you. As a nurse, you are likely to remember the nursing members of the interview team most easily by their titles or roles when they are introduced.

Most interview teams are aware of the anxiety aroused when being interviewed by a team and apply a variety of strategies to help you feel comfortable. If only printed name tags were included in their strategy, you would have it made!

Executive Career Search Services

Many trends affecting the health care industry, women in management, and leadership in nursing have created executive careers for nurses. As need for nurses as managers, senior administrators, and corporate executives emerges, organizations will expand their executive search services to obtain highly qualified applicants for these positions.

Executive search specialists, often called head hunters in the corporate world, market the organization to the candidate and the candidate to the organization. They have four main roles related to the candidate: recruiting, refining resumes, preparing for the interview, and negotiating salary. Their functions related to the organization are to search, recruit, provide background information, and schedule interviews. The executive search specialist negotiates specifics related to the position with both the organization and the candidate as the need arises.

Talking with corporate executive nurses and others who have had experiences with executive search services will help you gather information. The National League for Nursing provides nurse executive placement services to member agencies as well as continuing education and consultation services. If you receive a phone call from an executive search specialist, listen to what is being offered. If you are not interested, feel free to say so without obligation. You may be asked to recommend other candidates, and you should feel free to respond professionally. Should you recommend other colleagues, notify them so that they will not be surprised or feel obligated. If you are interested in the offer or in just finding out more about it, by all means follow through, as it may be the offer you have been awaiting.

Marketing Within an Organization

Marketing your expertise does not necessarily mean moving from one organization to another. It may mean repackaging your expertise to meet specifically identified needs within the same organization. It may also mean expanding your career to include more than one position. The results of your marketing efforts will reflect the extent to which you believe in yourself and the amount of energy you invest in convincing your potential employer that you are the person best suited for the position. For additional assistance on writing inquiry letters and resumes, see the bibliography at the end of the book.

Negotiating

Negotiating is an open communication process between individuals or between representatives of groups of individuals for the purpose of reaching an agreement. Are you a member of a committee or team that negotiates economic and general welfare issues for your organization? If so, do you apply these same skills to situations important to you in managing your career? If you have not had negotiating experience as a member of a committee or team, do you effectively communicate with others in your work setting to effect agreements that are beneficial to you and the organization? Do you feel comfortable negotiating for modifications to your position within an organization? How do you use negotiating skills when interviewing for new positions? Some examples of how nurses use negotiating skills to manage careers are provided here.

Anna and Jan are negotiators who bargain for their time and talent contributions in relation to their organizations'. Anna's case is one of initial reticence and illustrates her involvement with a coach that resulted in a successful outcome. Jan, who is experienced in representing other nurses in negotiating economic and general welfare issues, successfully transferred his skills to his own career management.

Case Example: Anna

Anna's formal introduction to the rules of negotiating was in a relationship with a superior. She was reluctant to cultivate and use negotiating skills, believing herself to be a nonargumentative person who avoided conflict. Two years of observing her superior led to some self-study and reassessment of her stance. Anna began to practice strategies to accomplish her goals. She used facts to support her view of flexible hours as optimal for her contribution to the organization in the face of specific time limits and fixed salaries. Anna and her superior negotiated an agreement to their mutual benefit.

Case Example: Jan

Jan was offered a position by an institution where, despite placement on the salary scale commensurate with organizational policy, his salary would be less than in his previous position. Since he was sure of his career goal, confident that he was the best person for the job, and had already convinced the organization of these facts, Jan negotiated a trade-off (a mutually agreed on option) to work a 4-day week to counterbalance financial remuneration in proportion to his contribution.

Resources that specify negotiating techniques are included in the Bibliography at the end of the book for more in-depth review and application. The following section on negotiating agreements is arranged in four subsections: assessment, planning, implementation, and evaluation. Each subsection contains key components for successfully negotiating agreements that may be applied to managing your nursing career. Exercises included in each subsection are an opportunity to assess your attitudes, knowledge, and skills related to negotiating.

Assessment.   The results of the assessment process should help you state for yourself what you want to accomplish from negotiation and explore your negotiating attitudes, knowledge, and skills. In Chapters 6 and 7 you specified preferred nursing options and career goals. Think of your results from exercises in those chapters and determine the extent to which you want to accomplish them. Do you want them badly enough to invest whatever it takes to get them, or do you want them only enough to get them with a safe investment? Your answers to these questions will help shape your expectations. Your expectations are based on the extent to which you know what you want and what you are willing to do to get it. List your expectations in the space provided here.

_____

_____

_____

_____

Exercise 9–6   Negotiating Assessment

This exercise will help you assess your attitudes, knowledge, and skills related to negotiating agreements important to your career. Keeping in mind what

you want and what you are willing to do to achieve what you want, respond
to the following questions by placing a check mark in the appropriate
column related to frequency.

	Frequency			
Question	*Often*	*Sometimes*	*Rarely*	*Never*

1. Do you make yourself available to listen to problems of those with whom you work (peers, subordinates, and superiors)?

2. Do you help others look at all options when discussing problems?

3. Do you believe that the give-and-take in problem-solving communication with others in your organization is effective?

4. Do you try to see problems and options from others' point(s) of view?

5. Are you firm in maintaining the focus of communication on main themes?

6. Are you aware of the importance of the following when communicating with others?

   a. Timing (punctuality and reasonable duration)

   b. Setting (optimal comfort)

   c. Specific questions (to clarify or validate information)

   d. General questions (to gather information)

   e. Nonverbal cues (eye contact, voice quality, body movements)

   f. Space (physical distance between persons who are communicating)

   g. Style (expressions of individual essence, eg, competitive, responsive, positive, collaborative, compliant, distant, negative)

   h. Feedback (exchanging the meanings of messages)

   i. Active listening (hearing, evaluating, predicting, reviewing, and remembering key ideas)

   j. Silence (ability to allow appropriate periods without spoken communication, eg, while you or others formulate thoughts into words)

Interpretation

Items 1, 2, 4, and 5 assess your open communication skills. If you use them often, you are probably skilled in winning when negotiating agreements. If you rarely or never use them and would like to develop them, the following strategies may help.

First, identify a hypothetical situation related to your career that requires using these skills. If you prefer to practice alone, use visualization. Allow yourself to experience the feelings that result from doing this. Then put yourself in the other person's place and visualize the range of possible responses. If you would like another person's input, try role playing. Discuss your and the other's perceptions of the verbal and nonverbal messages communicated. Another strategy is to consult a mentor or role model about ways to improve these skills. Additionally, you may want to read some of the references at the end of this chapter, which include specific techniques.

Item 3 assesses your attitude about the use of open communication in your organization. If your response to this item is rarely or never, on what information do you base your belief? Accurate information about those with whom you openly communicate and the extent to which they mirror the organization's philosophy is a key advantage. Attempting to negotiate without sufficient information is like attempting to take care of a client postoperatively without knowing what surgery was performed. If you feel that your information reservoir is adequate, you may benefit from reassessing your attitude toward the change process (see bibliography at the end of the book), the philosophy of your organization, or both.

An attitude of give-and-take in problem-solving communication is an aspect of openness essential for vitality, growth, and change. It requires that you communicate your perceptions and data about an experience or situation. Furthermore, it requires that the other person communicate his or her perceptions and data. Arriving at an agreement requires mutual respect and openness to changing views; it will take time, patience, and energy. Only you can assess your feelings about the extent of your investment in accomplishing what is important to managing your career. Remember, the extent of your success in negotiating reflects the extent of your expectations. High expectations yield moderate results; low expectations yield lower results.

Items 6a–6j assess your knowledge of components essential for effective negotiation. Since a moderate working knowledge of each element is important, responses of "often" and "sometimes" to all 10 validate your knowledge. Also think of them as skills and reassess the frequency with which you apply them. A response of "rarely" or "never" to any one item indicates the need for focusing on that area using strategies that best suit you.

Planning.   Now that you know what you want, the extent to which you want it, and the knowledge, skills, and attitudes needed for negotiating it, it is time to design a negotiating plan.

Exercise 9–7   Planning Negotiations

Respond to each of the following questions in the space provided.

1. What are all possible consequences for negotiating your career goal that you described earlier? List them.

_____

_____

_____

_____

2. Of these consequences, which are the best possible and least possible? What do you and others stand to gain? List in ranking order best possible to least possible consequences, and note your and others' gains in the appropriate columns.

A.	*Best possible*	*Your gains*	*Others' gains*
	_____	_____	_____
	_____	_____	_____
	_____	_____	_____
	_____	_____	_____
	_____	_____	_____
	_____	_____	_____

B.	*Least possible*	*Your gains*	*Others' gains*
	_____	_____	_____
	_____	_____	_____
	_____	_____	_____
	_____	_____	_____
	_____	_____	_____

(Bottom line)

3. What is the optimum strategy for accomplishing the best possible results?

_____

Interpretation

With your negotiation plan in mind, discuss options, trade-offs, and the bottom line based on your awareness of what is important to your career. Your options are derived from items 2A and 2B and should illustrate mutual gains. Your bottom line is the least possible option you will accept. It should be the last item in column 2B. Your trade-off is the adaptation of any of your options to a point of mutual agreement acceptable to you and the other person. It is often wise to agree to a trade-off on a trial or temporary basis. For example, "I'm willing to try _____ for three months, then I'd like us to reevaluate and discuss it further." It is also wise that your options, bottom line, and trade-off be based on objective, observable, or measurable criteria (for example, enhanced client satisfaction with the delivery of client care services, increased enrollment of nursing students, enhanced job satisfaction, or decreased employee turnover).

Implementation. With a clear goal and comprehensive plan, you are ready to use your strategy to accomplish your goal. Then, if necessary, try other options, trade-off, or the bottom line. In order to do this successfully, use your knowledge and skills of open communication with an attitude of high expectation and self-confidence. You are encouraged to write your plan, visualize yourself implementing it, and experience the feelings that result. You may choose to rehearse it with another person. Once you are ready, do it!

Evaluation. The evaluation of the extent to which your negotiation is successful depends on how you feel and several other criteria. Exercise 9–8 helps you examine the elements of evaluation.

Exercise 9–8   Evaluating Negotiations

Respond to each of the following questions in the space provided.

1. How do you feel now that you have tried negotiating?

   a. What aspects of the process made you feel good about you?

   _____

   _____

   b. What were areas in which you felt least prepared?

   _____

   _____

   c. To what extent are you satisfied with the outcome?

      _____ Highly satisfied

      _____ Satisfied

      _____ Ambivalent

      _____ Dissatisfied

      _____ Disappointed

      _____ Other (please write in) _____

2. If you feel ambivalent or dissatisfied, to what do you attribute these feelings?

   _____

   _____

   a. Was your goal realistic? _____

   b. Did you feel confident in knowledge? _____ Skills? _____

   c. Do you feel that your image was one of self-confidence and high expectations?

   _____

3. If you feel disappointed about the outcome, can you visualize your disappointment as your unmet expectations?

   a. If so, what were your expectations specifically? _____

   _____

   b. In what ways were they unmet?

   _____

   _____

Considering the evaluation results, only you can decide on the next step. If you were successful, congratulations! If not, is your goal important enough to take what you have learned from this experience and reassess, replan, reimplement, and reevaluate it? Using career management strategies is a lifelong process of taking responsibility for the choices and direction of roles and activities associated with the work aspects of your life.

Networking

Networking was discussed in Chapter 4 as a means of gathering information. As a mode of exchange of essential or desired information it also is a key career management strategy. Through networking, you can either purposefully or inadvertently market your expertise. Nurses are increasingly discovering clues about available positions and career opportunities through networking. You may find networking opportunities in social groups, at conferences, conventions, or meetings, while traveling, and through follow-up with authors of print media. Increasingly in nursing, significant decisions emerge from networking during a meal, over a drink, and on the golf course, for example. Some networks spawn other networks; for example, it is not unusual for a new network to begin with the exchange of business cards or phone numbers.

Case Examples: Shana, Keith, and Lorna

Shana, a pediatric nurse practitioner, school nurse, and nursing instructor on short-term leave from her teaching position, was referred to her present employer for a position as an occupational nurse through spontaneous networking with a former classmate at a social gathering. Shana loves the freedom and flexibility of her new position, which she now combines with short-term, part-time teaching.

Keith, a new graduate, used networking opportunities he discovered during an informational interview to follow-up on leads for a position as a nurse with the Peace Corps in Jamaica.

Lorna was 46 years old and recently divorced when an opportunity for a challenging change in her lifestyle and nursing career resulted from networking during a golf tournament. She is now working as a self-employed copyeditor and scriptwriter for a west coast medical media firm while studying journalism at a local university.

Successful career management through networking is not restricted to finding or changing positions. Other examples include consultation leads, publishing or research opportunities, and the exploration of dilemmas you are experiencing in your current position or institution.

Although networking strategies are not new, they are being increasingly emphasized in corporate media. According to John Naisbitt (1981), "the failure of hierarchies to solve society's problems forced people to talk to one another and that was the beginning of networks." Table 9–3 lists some advantages of networking, and Table 9–4 lists disadvantages.

Successful strategies depend on visibility (high or low profile according to individual preference), assertiveness, persistence, and sensitivity. The range of benefits and opportunities of effective networking in managing your career are endless.

TABLE 9–3   Advantages of Networking

Networking accomplishes the following:
1. Builds support systems
2. Fosters self-help
3. Improves productivity and work life
4. Encourages liaisons between clusters of like-minded individuals with mutually held ideas and values
5. Fosters a sense of belonging
6. Expedites the exchange of information
7. Encourages the refinement of loosely held ideas
8. Generates other networks
9. Fosters egalitarianism rather than elitism
10. Enhances both personal and professional development
11. Liberates creativity and innovation
12. Emphasizes cooperation and de-emphasizes competition

TABLE 9–4   Disadvantages of Networking

Negative consequences of networking include the following:
1. Overextension of personal resources
2. Splintering of efforts
3. Dilution of initiative
4. Diffusion of purpose
5. Conflict of values
6. Increased egocentrism and decreased altruism
7. Overdependence on others
8. Clouding of foresight
9. Feeling used
10. Feeling inadequate
11. Elitism rather than egalitarianism
12. Competition rather than cooperation

Managing Your Career in Nursing

The process of managing your career in nursing is lifelong, continuing to be useful to you in various stages of your personal and professional growth. Knowing why career management in nursing is important provides you with sound rationale for developing a career perspective. A career perspective guides you in applying a career management framework, which includes gathering data about yourself, nursing options, and trends and identifying personal, professional, and career goals. The use of career management processes and strategies illuminates your career path and insures control of your career future.

References

Girdano D, Everly G: *Controlling Stress and Tension: A Holistic Approach.* Englewood Cliffs, NJ: Prentice-Hall, 1979.

Moorpark College Counseling Staff: *Career and Life Planning,* p. 71. Moorpark, CA: Moorpark College Counseling, 1979.

Naisbitt J: *Megatrends.* New York: Warner Books, 1982.

Potter B: *Beating Job Burnout.* San Francisco: Harbor Publishing, 1980.

Selye H: *The Stress of Life.* New York: McGraw-Hill, 1978.

Smythe E: *Surviving Nursing.* Menlo Park, CA: Addison-Wesley, 1984.

Tubesing D: *Stress Skills.* Oakbrook, IL: Whole Person Associates, 1979.

Webster's New World Dictionary, 2nd ed., pp. 115; 868; 1293; 1431. New York: Simon and Schuster, 1984.

Appendix

Sample Inquiry Letter

August 6, 1984

Marie Craig, RN, MS
Director of Nursing
Hillview Medical Center
3250 Hillview Dr
Hillview, CA 91113

Dear Ms. Craig:

I am interested in a position on your staff as a unit coordinator for hospitalized older adults. I am currently Assistant Unit Coordinator for a 45-bed, eight-member staff unit for interdisciplinary care to hospitalized older adults in San Diego. I am a graduate of Los Angeles River College in Los Angeles. In December 1984, I will complete requirements for my Bachelor of Science degree in nursing from the California State University Consortium, Long Beach. During my 2 years of professional experience as a staff nurse at Memorial Hospital, San Diego, I planned, implemented, and evaluated nursing care of older adults with recurring illness problems.

I read of the expansion of your inpatient services to older adults in the *Los Angeles Times* in July. According to the article, you plan to admit clients to the new wing soon after January 1985. I will be relocating to the Hillview area in late December 1984. At your earliest convenience, I would like to visit Hillview Medical Center and explore with you potential openings for such a position. I have enclosed a resume for your information. You may reach me by phone at home until 3 pm, (604)753-3375, or at Memorial Hospital, Unit D, after 4 pm, (604)735-5733 Ext 2003. I look forward to hearing from you.

Sincerely yours,

Stacey Monte, RN

Curriculum Vitae Sample

Michelle Yvette Boyd
Project Coordinator
Oak College School of Nursing
Oak Park, CA 94537
(415)659-6906

1640 Hays Lane
Menlo, CA 94033
(415)856-0524

Education

1958	BSN, Orleans University, New Orleans, LA
1966	MS, University of California
1978	EdD, Forrest University, Forrest Hill, FL

Experience

8/63–7/65	Staff Nurse, Psychiatry, VA Hospital, Altos, CA
8/65–8/66	Head Nurse, Psychiatry, VA Hospital, Altos, CA
9/66–12/69	Supervisor, Psychiatry, VA Hospital, Altos, CA
1/70–7/74	Psychiatric Liaison Nurse, Memorial Medical Center, San Diego, CA
9/74–8/76	Instructor, Nursing Department, Marshall Community College, Marshall, CA
9/76–7/80	Assistant Director, Nursing Department, Marshall Community College, Marshall, CA
8/80–6/82	Coordinator, Nursing Department, Carver Community College, Carver, CA
8/82–present	Project Coordinator, Oak College, Oak Park, CA

Honors

1978	Recipient, Outstanding Graduate Award, Forrest University

Professional Memberships

American Nurses' Association

California League for Nursing

California Nurses' Association

National League for Nursing

Sigma Theta Tau—Alpha Eta Chapter

Western Society for Research in Nursing Education

Publications

Boyd MY: Time perception in hospitalized patients with diagnosis of chronic schizophrenia. *J Psychiatr Nurs* (April/May) 1968; 1(2):68–72.

Boyd MY: The integration of therapeutic communication into community college nursing curricula. *J Nurs Educ* (Sept) 1974; 2(3):34–37.

Arsen JB, Boyd MY: Leadership and management styles in community college nursing programs. *J Nurse Educ* (Nov) 1980; 4(3):44–49.

Boyd MY, Carter BJ: Graduate education for nurses from ethnic groups traditionally underrepresented in higher education: A success model. *Nursing Forum* (Jan/Feb) 1983; 2(1):26–29.

Boyd MY, Jones KC, Smith MD: *Career Counseling for Nurses by Nurses.* Reading, MA: Addison-Wesley, 1983.

Boyd MY: Validating the NLN competency statements. Paper presented by M. Boyd and S. Sousa at the Second Annual Conference of The Society for Research in Nursing Education, San Francisco, January 1983. Abstracted in *Nurs Res* (Oct) 1983; 1(4):12.

Boyd MY: Who's in the real world, service or education? Paper presented by M. Boyd at the First Annual Convention of the California League for Nursing, Sacramento, CA, March 1983.

Creative Resume Sample

Resume

Demographic Data

Name	Michelle Yvette Boyd, RN, EdD
Home Address	1640 Hayes Lane
and Telephone	Menlo, CA 94033
	(415)856-0524
Employer Address	Oak College
and Telephone	43600 Mission Blvd
	Oak Park, CA 94537
	(415)659-6906
RN License Number	165348; Expiration date 5/31/88

Credentials

1973	Life credential, Community college instructor: Nursing
1975	Life credential, Community college counselor
1976	Life credential, Community college supervisor

Education

1984	Certificate in Human Resource Management, University of California, Santa Cruz, CA
1978	EdD Forrest University, Forrest Hill, FL, Higher education
1966	MS, University of California
1958	BSN, Orleans University, New Orleans, LA

Professional Experience

8/82-present	Project Coordinator, Oak College, Oak Park, CA
8/80–6/82	Coordinator, Nursing Department, Carver Community College, Carver, CA
9/76–7/80	Assistant Director, Nursing Department, Marshall Community College, Marshall, CA
9/74–8/76	Instructor, Nursing Department, Marshall Community College, Marshall, CA

1/70–7/74	Psychiatric Liaison Nurse, Memorial Medical Center, San Diego, CA
9/66–12/69	Supervisor, Psychiatry, VA Hospital, Altos, CA
8/65–8/66	Head Nurse, Psychiatry, VA Hospital, Altos, CA
8/63–7/65	Staff Nurse, Psychiatry, VA Hospital, Altos, CA

Professional Publications and Presentations

Boyd MY: The integration of therapeutic communication into community college nursing curricula, *J Nurs Educ* (Sept) 1974; 2(3):34–37.

Arsen JB, Boyd MY: Leadership and management styles in community college nursing programs, *J Nurse Educ* (Nov) 1980; 4(3):44–49.

Boyd MY, Carter BJ: Graduate education for nurses from ethnic groups traditionally underrepresented in higher education: A success model. *Nurs Forum* (Jan/Feb) 1983; 2(1):26–29.

Boyd MY, Jones KC, Smith MD: *Career Counseling for Nurses by Nurses.* Reading, MA: Addison-Wesley, 1983.

Continuing Education

7/1/83–7/14/83	Clinical performance in nursing examinations training session, Forrest University, Forrest Hill, FL

Memberships

American Nurses' Association

California League for Nursing

California Nurses' Association

National League for Nursing

Western Society for Research in Nursing Education

References available on request

Functional Resume Sample

Resume

9/84

Stacey Monte
180 Spruce Dr
Encinitas, CA 91112
Home Phone: (604)753-3375

Professional Objective:	Managing client care for hospitalized older adults
Experience:	
1982–1984	Memorial Hospital, San Diego, CA Staff Nurse Gerontopsychology Planned, implemented, and evaluated nursing care of older adults with recurring illness problems.
1984–present	Memorial Hospital, San Diego Assistant Unit Coordinator Coordinate scheduling, nursing care planning, and care for a staff of eight, including three nurses, on the 4 PM to midnight shift. Client load: 30 to 45 older adults with recurring illness problems.
Education:	
1982	Los Angeles River College, Van Nuys, CA Associate in Science degree
1983	California State University Consortium, Long Beach Bachelor of Science in nursing program
Continuing Education:	
1/2/83	Memorial Hospital, San Diego, CA Health care delivery models for hospitalized older adults
8/5/83	An interdisciplinary approach to holistic care for chronically ill older adults
6/5/84	Cost-effective patient care planning
References:	

Professional and personal references available on request.

Sample Thank You Letter Following an Interview

September 16, 1984

Marie Craig, RN, MS
Director of Nursing
Hillview Medical Center
3250 Hillview Dr
Hillview, CA 91113

Dear Ms. Craig:

Thank you for the opportunity to interview with you, Mr. Gray, Personnel Officer, and Ms. Greene, Staff Coordinator, on September 15. I am enthusiastic about the opportunities available at Hillview Medical Center in interdisciplinary care of hospitalized older adults. I enjoyed the tour of the new wing and would welcome an opportunity to be involved with the process of setting it up to receive patients in January 1985.

I look forward to a favorable response from your screening committee.

Sincerely yours,

Stacey Monte, RN

Bibliography

Career Planning and Management

General

Arbeiter S: Forty million Americans in career transition, the need for information. Final Report. Princeton, NJ: College Entrance Exam Board, 1978.

Bott P et al: It's time to shift gears from career planning to life planning. *Training/HRD* 1980; 17:74.

Buskirk R: *Your Career: How to Plan, Manage, Change it.* Boston: C. B. Publishing, 1980.

Erickson K: A model for developing and operating an adult peer guidance center. Circa, Arizona Center for Educational Research and Development, Arizona University at Tuscon, College of Education (Ed. 160.917), 1978.

Henderson F: *A life-centered, competency-based approach to career guidance, program planning and personal counseling for students interested in nursing and health-related careers,* Unpublished major applied research project. Nova University, Fort Lauderdale, FL, 1978.

Knowdell R: The implementation of career life planning program in an industrial setting. Paper presented June 1978, Annual Conference of American Society of Engineer Education, British Columbia, 1978.

London M, Stumpf S: *Managing Careers.* Reading, MA: Addison-Wesley, 1982.

Mannebach A: Theories of career development and occupational choice. Paper presented April 1979, American Educational Research Association, (Ed. 167.833), 1979.

Michelozzi B: *Coming Alive from 9 to 5.* Palo Alto: Mayfield, 1980.

Morre E, Miller T: Comprehensive career guidance. Post-secondary and adult programs and model. University of Missouri, Columbia, College of Education, 1977.

Perry W: *Forms of Intellectual and Ethical Development in the College Years, a Scheme.* San Francisco: Holt, Rinehart and Winston, 1970.

Robbins P: *Successful Midlife Career Change: Self-understanding and Strategies for Action.* New York: Amacom, 1978.

Sayles L, Strauss G: *Managing Human Resources.* Englewood Cliffs, NJ: Prentice Hall, 1981.

Vetter L, et al.: Career planning programs for women employees: a national survey. Center for Research in Vocational Education, Ohio State University, Columbus. Research and Development Series 135 (Ed. 170.600), 1977.

Wanous J: *Organizational Entry*. Reading, MA: Addison-Wesley, 1980.

Nursing

Anastas L: *Your Career in Nursing*. New York: National League for Nurses, 1984.

Donley R: Nursing careerists. *Imprint* 1985; 31(5):8–11.

Dunkelberger J, Aadland S: Expectations and attainment of nursing careers. *Nurs Res* 1985; 33(4):235–240.

Flaherty M: On being fully alive as a person and as a nurse. *Nurs Management* 1983; 14(7):50–51.

Friss L: An expanded conceptualization of job satisfaction and career style. *Nurs Leadership* 1981; 4(4):13–22.

Garrett C: Adult women entering nursing: motivational factors and personality orientations. Columbia University, Teachers College. Dissertation Abstracts International, (May) 1984; 44(11):

Hale M: Future planning: occupation and career choices. *Imprint* (Feb) 1982; 29:14.

Keough G: The need for nursing career development. *J Contin Educ Nurs*, 8:(5&6).

Kleinknecht M et al: Assisting nurses toward professional growth: a career development model. *J Nurs Admin* (July/Aug) 1982; 12:30–36.

Lolito M, Kostenbauer J: *Advance: The Nurses Guide to Success in Today's Job Market*. Boston: Little Brown, 1981

London F: Why choose nursing? *Am J Nurs* (Jan) 1985; 85:114.

Nowick J, Gindel C: *Career Planning in Nursing*. Philadelphia: Lippincott, 1984.

Price J, Randolph G: Career trajectory in nursing: the randice approach. *Nurs Success* (March/April) 1984; 1:21–25.

Robinson A: Making a career choice: think twice. *Imprint* (Sept) 1979; 26(3):10–12.

Robinson-Smith G: Alternate careers in nursing. *Imprint* (Dec) 1984; 30(5):23–24.

Scaffer M, Moody Y: A model for career development. *J Nurs Educ* 1980; 19(8):42–46.

Schwartz I: Try this model HRD system: it matches individual and organizational goals. *Training/HRD* (Nov) 1979; 16:52–56.

Scott P: Executive career planning. *Nurs Econ* (Jan/Feb) 1984; 2:58–63.

Smith MM: Career development in nursing: an individual and professional responsibility. *Nurs Outlook* (Feb) 1982; 30(2):128–131.

Swansburg R, Swansburg P: *Strategic Career Planning and Development for Nurses.* Rockville, MD: Aspen Pub., 1984.

The New Nurse—A Career for All Reasons. NY: National League for Nursing, 1982.

The New Nurse—A Career for All Reasons . . . and All People. NY: National League for Nursing, 1982.

The New Nurse—A Career for All Reasons (Counselor's/teacher's guide). NY: National League for Nursing, 1982.

The New Nurse—A Career to Turn to and Return To. NY: National League For Nursing, 1982

Career and Self

Crego M, Tymchyshyn P, Lewis J: *Introduction to Independent Learning Module 2: Learning and Lifestyle Management.* Statewide Nursing Program, the Consortium of the California State University, Long Beach, 1984.

Kangas J, Solomon G: *The Psychology of Strength.* Englewood Cliffs, NJ: Prentice-Hall, 1975.

Keeton M et al: *Experiential Learning: Rationale Characteristics and Assessment,* pp. 62–106. San Francisco: Jossey-Bass, 1977.

Levenstein A: What they want from work. *Nurs Management* 1983; 14(6):42–43.

Mandelkorn P: *To Know Your Self: The Essential Teaching of Swami Satchidananda.* New York: Anchor Press, 1978.

Putt A: *General Systems Theory Applied to Nursing.* Boston: Little Brown, 1978.

Reres M: Self-assessment and career choice. *Imprint* (March) 1979; 26(3):13–16.

Robinson A: Career choice by lifestyle—the better way. *Imprint* 1980; 27(4):7–8.

Sangiuliano I: *In Her Time.* New York: William Morrow, 1978.

Schiffman M: *Self Therapy: Techniques for Personal Growth.* Menlo Park, CA: Self Therapy Press, 1967.

Career Strategies

Brallier L: *Transition and Transformation: Successfully Managing Stress.* Los Altos, CA: National Nursing Review, 1982.

Bruce G: An evaluation of marketing in nursing. *Stanford Nurse* (Spring) 1984;11–13.

Duncan J, Partridge R: Peer pals: overcoming the obstacles to leadership development. *Nurs Leadership* 1980; 3(2):18–21.

Eliopoulos C: Selling a positive image builds demand. *Nurs Management* 1985; 14(4):23–30.

Filoroma T: Career pathing (or finding a job). *Imprint* 1985;31:12–17.

Fisher R, Ury W: *Getting to Yes.* Boston: Houghton Mifflin, 1981.

Fleischer S, Rosenbaum B: Job market realities for the health care professional. Presented to Management Career Services at California League for Nursing Convention, May 24, 1984. Sacramento, CA.

Illich J: *Power Negotiating Strategies for Winning in Life and in Business.* Menlo Park, CA: Addison-Wesley, 1980.

Illich J, Jones B: *Successful Negotiating Skills for Women.* Reading, MA: Addison-Wesley, 1981.

Jackson J: *The Whole Nurse Catalog.* Philadelphia: Saunders, 1980.

Josefowitz N: *Paths to Power.* Reading, MA: Addison-Wesley, 1980.

Kalisch B, Kalisch P: Nursing image: the tv news picture. *Nurs Management* 1985; 16(4):39–48.

Marriner A: Time management for career development. *Nurs Success Today* 1984; 1(2):4–7.

May K, Melies A, Winstead-Fry P: Mentorship for scholarliness: opportunities and dilemmas. *Nurs Outlook* (Jan) 1982; 30(1):22–28.

Meisenhelder J: Networking and nursing. *Image* 1982; 410(3):77–80.

Miller D: *Personal Vitality.* Reading, MA: Addison-Wesley, 1977.

Newcomb J, Murphey P: The curriculum vitae—what it is and what it is not. *Nurs Outlook* (Sept) 1979;27:580–583.

Nurse Executive Placement Service (brochure). NY: National League for Nursing.

Parker M: How to write your resume. *Am J Nurs* 1979; 79(10):1739–1741.

Pilette P: Mentoring: an encounter of the leadership kind. *Nurs Leadership* 1980; 3(2):22–26.

Resume Preparation Manual—A Step by Step Guide for Women. New York: Catalyst, 1976.

Stanton M: Patient and health education: lessons for the market place. *Nurs Management* 1985; 16(4):28–30.

Trygstad J, Morris K: Entry into practice: a career entry guide for nurses. *Imprint* 1980; 27(4):19–23.

Warschaw T: *Winning by Negotiation.* New York: Berkeley Books, 1980.

Information Collection

Beasley S: Anatomy of a grants process. *Grantmanship Center News* (May–Aug) 1978; 4:62–78.

Center for women and work: Keeping a job journal. *The Career Development Seminar for Women Office Workers.* Washington, DC: National Institute for Work and Learning, 1980.

Saba V, Skapik K: Nursing information center. *Am J Nurs* (Jan) 1979; 79: 86–87.

Smith M, Felix J: *A Directory of Nursing-Related Data Sources.* Boulder, CO: National Center for Higher Education Management Systems, Western Interstate Commission for Higher Education, 1977.

Stoia J: Nursing instruction: can data base searching enhance the practice? A guide to the novice user. *J Nurs Educ* 1983; 22(2):74–79.

Taylor S: How to search the literature. *Am J Nurs* 1974; 74(8):1457–1459.

US Department of Health and Health Services: *Nursing Personnel* (Sourcebook). USDHHS Publication No. (HRA)18:21, 1981.

Nursing Options

Adam E: *To Be a Nurse.* Philadelphia: Saunders, 1980.

ANA Commission on Nursing Research: *Research in Nursing: Toward a Science of Health Care.* Kansas City, MO: American Nurses' Association, 1976.

ANA Commission on Nursing Services: A guide for nurses considering a career move in nursing administration. Kansas City, MO: American Nurses' Association Publication No. N.S.-26 3M, 1979.

Archer S, Fleshman R: Community health nursing: A typology of practice. *Nurs Outlook* 1978; 23(6):358–364.

Aydelotte M: Part 1: A survey of nursing service administrators. *Hospitals* 1984; 58(11):94–100.

Calvecchio R: Direct patient care: a viable career choice? *J Nurs Admin* 1982; 12(7):17–22.

Calvecchio R, Tescher B, Scalzi C: A clinical ladder for nursing practice. *J Nurs Admin* 1974; 4(5):54–58.

Campbell C: Special clinics: The microbe hunters . . . nursing patients with sexually transmitted diseases. *Nurs Mirror* (June) 1982; 154:48.

Choi M: Nurses as co-providers of primary health care. *Nurs Outlook* (Sept) 1981; 29(9):519–521.

Colerick E et al: Evaluation of the clinical nurse specialist role: development and implementation of a dual purpose framework. *Nurs Leadership* (Sept) 1980; 3:26–34.

Deckert B et al: Clinical ladders. *Nurs Management* 1984; 15(3):54–56; 58–62.

Fawcett J: Theory: basis for the study and practice of nursing education. *J Nurs Educ* 1985; 24(6):226–229.

Fine R: Health information brokers . . . matching the needs of client-patients with the resources of the health care system. *Nurs Management* (June) 1982; 13:39–40.

Ford L: A nurse for all settings: the nurse practitioner. *Nurs Outlook* (Aug) 1979; 27:516–521.

Ganong J, Ganong W: *Cases in Nursing Management.* Rockville, MD: Aspen, 1979.

Guide to nursing specialities from anesthesia to—would you believe?—zoology. *Nurs '78* 1978; 8(11): (Oct) 57–64; (Nov) 49–56.

Guidelines in educational preparation and competencies of the school nurse practitioner. *J School Health* 1978; 48(5):265–268.

Hall B, Mitsunaga B, de Tornyay R: Deans of nursing: changing socialization patterns. *Nurs Outlook* 1981; 29(2):92–95.

Jacox A, Norris C: *Organizing for Independent Nursing Practice.* New York: Appleton-Century-Crofts, 1977.

Kiker M: Characteristics of an effective teacher. *Nurs Outlook* 1973; 21:721–723.

Koch M: Use your nursing experience in product manufacturing: Become a nurse consultant in industry. *Nurs '79* (July) 1979; 9:72–73.

Kohnke M: *Case for Consultation in Nursing.* New York: Wiley, 1978.

Lange F: Multifaceted role of the nurse consultant. *J Nurs Educ* 1979; 18(9):30–34.

McMurrey P: Toward a unique knowledge base in nursing. *Image* 1982; 14(1):12–15.

Nerone B: Profile of a nurse researcher. *Imprint* (Feb) 1982; 29:41.

Notter L: The case for nursing research. *Nurs Outlook* 23:760–763.

Parrish A: Mental handicap nursing: a labour of love. *Nurs Mirror* (Dec) 1981; 153:48.

Rotkovitch R: The head nurse as a first-line manager. *Health Care Supervisor* 1983; 1(4):14–28.

Rufo K: Termination of a successful internship program. *J Nurs Admin* 1984; 14(6):33–37.

Schultz H, Henry O, Sullivan J: *Nurse Practitioners USA.* Boston: Lexington, 1979.

Schultz H, Zielenzy M: Longitudinal study of nurse practitioners phase III. US Department of Health, Education, and Welfare Publication No. (HRA) (#80-2). US Government Printing Office, 1980.

Simmons R, Rosenthal J: Women's movement and the nurse practitioner's sense of role. *Nurs Outlook* 29:371–375.

Stevens B: *Nursing Theory: Analysis, Application, Evaluation.* Boston: Little, Brown, 1979.

Stevens B: *The Nurse as Executive.* Boston: Nursing Resources, 1980.

Stricklin R: The rural ED nurse—an expanded role. *J Emerg Nurs* 1980; 6(5): 54–56.

Sullivan E, Decker P: *Effective Management in Nursing.* Menlo Park, CA: Addison-Wesley, 1985.

Take the Extra Step . . . Become a Certified Nurse. Kansas City, MO: American Nurses' Association, 1983.

Wollatt B: Drug dependency nursing: one hundred lives in the balance. *Nurs Mirror* (July) 1982; 155:52.

Professional and Societal Issues

Bower F: *Women and Careers.* Paper presented at acceptance of Outstanding Professor award, San Jose State University, San Jose, CA, 1982.

Brooten D, Hayden L, Naylor M: *Leadership for Change: A Guide for the Frustrated Nurse.* New York: Van Nostrand Co., 1978.

Brown K, Perkins C: The savvy 60. *Savvy* 1985; 6:50–59.

Bullough B: Influences on role expansion. *Am J Nurs* (Sept) 1976; 76:1476–1481.

Cleland D: The cultural ambience of the matrix organization. *Management Review* (Nov) 1981; 25–39.

Cohen H: *The Nurse's Quest for a Professional Identity.* Menlo Park, CA: Addison-Wesley, 1981.

Diers D: A different field of energy: nurse power. *Nurs Outlook* (Jan) 1978; 26:51–55.

Flynn P, Miller M: *Current Perspectives in Nursing.* St. Louis: Mosby, 1980.

Gilligan C: *In a Different Voice.* Cambridge, MA: Harvard University Press, 1982.

Harragan B: *Games Mother Never Taught You: Corporate Gamesmanship for Women.* New York: Rawson Assoc., 1977.

Hennig M, Jardin A: *The Managerial Woman.* New York: Doubleday, 1977.

McCarthy P: Practice acts too broad says report. *AM Nurse* 1982; 14(2):1; 26.

Morical L: *Where's My Happy Ending? Women and the Myth of Having It All.* Menlo Park, CA: Addison-Wesley, 1984.

Mundinger M: *Autonomy in Nursing.* Germantown, MD: Aspen, 1980.

Porcino J: *Growing Older, Getting Better.* Menlo Park, CA: Addison-Wesley, 1983.

Simms L, Lindberg J: *The Nurse Person.* San Francisco: Harper & Row, 1978.

Smith GR: Nursing beyond the crossroads. *Nurs Outlook* (Sept) 1980; 28:540–545.

Stevens B: *Nursing Theory, Analysis, Application, Evaluation.* Boston: Little, Brown, 1979.

Whitman M: Toward a new psychology for nurses. *Nurs Outlook* (Jan) 1982; 30:48–52.

Role Transition and Stress

Astbury J, Yu V: Determinants of stress for staff in a neonatal intensive care unit. *Arch Dis Child* 1982; 57(2):108–111.

Christman L: Problems of role definition, the health care team. In: *Current perspectives in nursing,* pp. 15–23. Flynn B, Miller M (editors). St. Louis: Mosby, 1980.

Gentry W, Parkes K: Psychological stress in intensive care unit–nonintensive care unit nursing: a review of the past decade. *Heart Lung* 1982; 11(1):43–47.

Hiraki A, Parlocha P: *Returning to School, The RN to BSN Handbook.* Boston, MA: Little Brown, 1983.

Pollock S: The stress response. Psychological crises in critical care. *Crit Care Quart* 1984; 6(4):1–11.

Riger S, Galligan P: Women in management: an exploration of competing paradigms. *AM Psychol* 1980; 35(10):102–110.

Sarbin T, Allen V: Role theory. In: *Handbook of social psychology,* pp. 488–567. Lindzey G, Aronson E (editors). Reading, MA: Addison-Wesley, 1968.

Trends

Abu-Saad H: *Nursing a World View.* St. Louis: Mosby, 1979.

Aiken L, Gortner S (editors): *Nursing in the 1980s: Crises, Opportunities, Challenges.* Philadelphia: Lippincott, 1982.

Bullough V, Bullough B: *History, Trends, and Politics of Nursing.* Norwalk, CT: Appleton-Century-Crofts, 1984.

Chaska N (editor): *The Nursing Profession: A Time to Speak.* New York: McGraw-Hill, 1983.

Culler S, Van Veen Diagle A (editors): *The American Health Care System.* Chicago, IL: American Medical Association, 1984.

Curtin L: The decade ahead: five major issues. (Editorial) *Nurs Management* (Oct) 1985; 14:9–10.

DeCrosta T: Megatrends in nursing. *Nurs Life* (May/June) 1985; 5:18–21.

Delbecq A, Van De Ven A, Gustafson D: *Group Techniques for Program Planning: A Guide to Nominal and Delphi Techniques.* Glenview, IL: Scott Foresman, 1975.

Hawken P, Ogilvy J, Schwartz P: *Seven Tomorrows.* NY: Bantam Books, 1982

Health care in the 1980s. NY: National Leage for Nursing, 1979.

Health expenditure patterns in the United States and California. *Socieoecon Rep* (March/April) 1983; 23(2):1–6.

Hospital Statistics. Chicago, IL: American Hospital Association, 1984.

Kalisch B: The promise of power. *Nurs Outlook* (Jan) 1978; 26:42–46.

McCauley M: Health care trends and issues in the 1980s. *Cross-Ref Hum Resources Management* (Sept/Oct) 1981; 11:5–8.

McCormick K: Preparing nurses for the technologic future. *Nurs Health Care* 1983; 4(9):379–382.

Millman M: *Nursing Personnel and the Changing Health Care System.* Cambridge, MA: Ballinger, 1978.

New Directions for Nursing in the '80s. Kansas City, MO: American Nurses' Association, 1980.

Stolovitch H: Focus on the future: From delphi to delphi. *Viewpoints* 1976; 52(2):9–20.

Styles M: Dialogue across the decades. *Nurs Outlook* (Jan) 1978; 26:28–32.

US Department of Health and Human Services, National Center for Health Statistics: *Health, United States, 1983.* DHHS Publication No. (PHS) 84-1232. US Government Printing Office, 1983.

US Department of Health and Human Services, PHS: *Promoting Health/Preventing Disease: Objectives for the Nation.* US Government Printing Office, 1980.

Weil R, Tyson P: The 2001 prophecy quiz. *Omni* (April) 1985; 40; 90; 92; 94.

What the next 50 years will bring. *USNWR* (May 9) 1983; A 1–42.

Index